Strokes from the Master's Brush:

Walking Through the Stages of a Stroke

By Bill Smallman

For Doris

CreateSpace 2017

Strokes from the Master's Brush: Walking through the Stages of a Stroke.

By Bill Smallman

The back cover photo of Doris Smallman in therapy was taken by the author, and the photo of us in Meet the Author on p. 86 was taken in 2008.

The lyrics to the song *You Are Still Holy* are quoted in their entirety, as sung by Kim Hill in the CD *Arms of Mercy*, of StarSong Records (Sparrow Group) © 1998 Mercy Publishing. Thank you.

Printed in the United States of America by CreateSpace® of Amazon.Com, Inc.® and available from Amazon.Com and other fine booksellers.

ISBN-10: 1546731989
ISBN-13: 978-1546731986

CONTENTS

DEDICATION

To Doris

This is a story, a true story, Doris' story. We all hear about someone who had a stroke, and it seems remote and mysterious. We pray, thinking, "Too bad," and go on about our lives. But this stroke struck OUR family, and this time we could not say, "Too bad" and go back to normal living. There was a new normal. Doris is the heroine of this story, so as her loving husband of over 50 years I dedicate this little work to her, my heroine, my model of courage in adversity. She may have seemed frail, but a load of trouble works in some people as a load does in a truck: the springs get tough, and the treads grip the road more firmly, so we grind the gears and move ahead more slowly. She never quit.

We also can never forget those doctors with all the specialties that we needed, along with their nurses, therapists, and aides. We would love to go back to all of them to share the glow of all that they accomplished in their thankless daily care.

We are grateful for the medical professionals who read an earlier draft of this work and gave helpful comments. It is not a medical approach to strokes, but we wanted its non-technical descriptions to be accurate and helpful.

WHY THIS BOOK?

Aren't the bookstores already crowded with books on strokes? Every such book serves a different purpose. They stress medical, or social, or spiritual, or therapeutic dimensions related to the various dimensions of strokes.

This book intends to be a friendly conversation with families that are facing some such shattering experience for the first time. We have been there, and have survived a massive stroke. Just knowing that you are not alone is helpful, especially when you suddenly feel bereft and abandoned.

Your experience is not like ours, as every stroke is unique. But our experience shows the commonalities of our experiences. When something serious happens to us we lean on others who have been through it already. For America, life changed in the devastation of September 11, 2001, but for the Smallman family that hinge of history was July 20, 2002. All of life was transformed in an instant, and yet it goes on. Grieving goes on and on, but so do the grit and guts and the git-up-and-go that make life worthwhile.

We will speak freely of our walk with God as born-again Christians. That may or may not be part of your experience, but you can watch to see whether that is mere religious talk or is a lively foundational basis for a life of victory and growth. Come walk with us for a while and see. You'll see our pain and puzzlement, our common humanity. Jesus did NOT say to us, "Get up and walk" as He did to some back in His day among us. Our case is more like that of the Apostle Paul to whom He said, "My strength is revealed in [your] weakness."

You will read and hear many stroke stories, all different. Our story is reduced to **seven basic stages** as a framework. The day WILL come when your story will encourage others along.

The seven stages I have identified may not fit your case as if it were a universal template. But you will readily sense at which stage you entered your own struggle, and come along with us. These are sort of like the subtitles of seven of our chapters.

1. **The causes stack up.** What led to this stroke?
2. **What actually happens in a stroke?**
3. **First response: intensive care**
4. **The in-hospital therapy and training**
5. **Coming home to changes, and**
6. **Out-patient therapy**
7. **Caregivers step up; Building a new life**

Just a couple of days after Doris' stroke I began writing my **Diary of a Stroke.** It was not meant to be read, but to help ME sort out what was happening to us. Some people cry when overwhelmed. Some people drink to pretend it will all go away. Some people pray to find solace. I write. When I can squeeze a major tragedy into sentences the matter becomes, or seems to become, more manageable. And I needed to keep straight all of the details that were flashing by. Now that I am polishing up this short book that *Diary* is an invaluable resource. Doris has started to read it a couple of times, but it made her uncomfortable. Our daughter Margie said, "I had to live through all that, so why read about it?" Wise. So the point was never that it be read, but that it be written.

I have encouraged others who are so inclined to write out their thoughts and feelings as they go through their own adventure. Someday you will look back on it all as a distant memory, even as you deal with its permanent aftereffects.

So come along with us so you won't feel so alone in the agony of your own stroke. Or it might be some other traumatic brain injury from the highway or battlefield or sports arena. No two journeys back to a new normalcy are the same, but they all follow the same general pathway. Many of us have survived the trek, and you will too.

1.

HOW DID <u>THAT</u> HAPPEN?

Stage 1: Causes Stack Up

It was a dark and stormy night. Oops, wrong book. Sorry 'bout that, Snoopy. Our stunning experience occurred in broad daylight on a sunny July day, though it suddenly seemed like a dark and stormy night. What happened? Why do WE suffer when we are "the good guys?" Lightning strikes, but did it have to hit OUR home? Yes.

Adversity is a magnet which draws people together. This journal of the massive stroke which hit Doris Klett Smallman on July 20, 2002, is simply a ledger of the evidence of the reality of God's grace as metered out through His people. Here is an outline of our medical and spiritual journey through deep waters when we could not see if there was an "other side" to come out on, but were confident that our Shepherd would "lead us beside still waters" in His time. We invite you to walk through it all with us, especially if you are reeling with grief of your own. Think of this little book as a conversation with friends who have been there, done that, and survived successfully. You can too. Come on along, pain and all.

Let's back up and set the stage, years in the past.

Watch the parade going down Main Street in Lombard, Illinois, just twenty miles straight west of Chicago. On a clear day (and they did have them back then) you could get a shadowy glimpse of the tall skyscrapers that crowded along Lake Michigan. In that fancy parade was Doris Klett, the Maytag

Queen in the simple float showing off the fancy appliances from her daddy's little store in the center of town. It was the Lilac Village at its best, and being Queen for a Day was a delight for a cute eight year old girl bursting with promise. Her two big brothers Bob and Don got to drive the car that pulled the float through town as the people cheered. You'll have to imagine that in black & white since it was before color TV.

The parade passed near the Lombard Bible Church that Doris' parents had helped to establish along with other families. It was through the children's ministries of that church that Doris called on the name of the Lord and began her spiritual pilgrimage. Wilbur and Betty Klett wanted their children to honor the Lord throughout their lives. They provided a wonderful launching pad for personal growth and useful service, a home that was loving and stable, granted the normal range of human ups and downs.

Sometime during those early years Doris came down with a bout of rheumatic fever as was more common in the 1940s. Little did anyone suspect the impact that those bothersome days of high fever would have on her adult life decades later. Mom Klett rubbed her with cool cloths and with prayer, seeking some comfort for her ailing child, until the fever finally broke and health was restored. For a while.

We fast forward through high school training in secretarial skills and summer jobs in the offices of engineering companies in Chicago. The "Roarin' Elgin" commuter train (OK, of the Aurora and Elgin line) breezed back and forth from Lombard's passenger station to Chicago.

Then she was off to college at John Brown University in Siloam Springs, Arkansas, where her brother Don was studying Architectural Design. There she met Bill Smallman who had come from Wheaton, Maryland, to study Mechanical Engineering. (I, your invisible narrator, am that fortunate man.)

As we found each other, there were common interests in serving God, and a shared sense of God's calling into missionary ministry. We graduated in May of 1962 full of normal dreams and aspirations and married that summer. Our first home was in southern California where I worked as an aerospace design engineer and also attended seminary. After pastoral experience in the Chicago area we joined Baptist Mid-Missions (Cleveland, Ohio) and took off for Manaus, Amazonas, Brazil, which was home for the decade of the 1970s. So our son David and daughter Margie got to grow up in Brazil, being five and three years old when we arrived early on a hot morning in August of 1970. It was our eighth wedding anniversary!

This whirlwind biographical sketch allows us to pick up the threads of Doris' health issues. There were rumors that the Amazon Valley tends to be hot and humid, and we can verify from our first-hand experience that it is true, especially the high humidity. We were in Manaus, the state capital of Amazonas, so there was air conditioning here and there (including our bedroom) even back then.

In that oppressive wet heat Doris began to have odd sensations in her heart after a couple of years. A mission colleague who is a nurse suspected Doris had atrial fibrillation, and took us to a cardiologist who lived right on our street. The occasional irregular heartbeat came on with times of stress, and was not to be ignored. The doctor tried this and that medication to find just the right medication in the right dosage to maintain cardiac regularity.

Since Doris was flying to the States to celebrate her parents' fiftieth wedding anniversary, the doctor suggested a cardiac workup there where more sophisticated monitoring equipment was readily available. And so she did. On our next visit to the cardiologist after that trip he said, "Before I see the report, let me tell you what I think is the problem." He explained that she may have had rheumatic fever as a child, and suffered some permanent damage to the mitral valve of the heart that has provoked the occasional arrhythmia. We just stared at each other in amazement.

Bingo! He was right on target. We felt all the more confident in him seeing that he could make an accurate diagnosis on the basis of limited testing but good training and intuition. The doc was also glad that the cardiologist in the States had tried yet another medication for regulating her pulse (that did not work) since that was the medicine he was going to try next. And the next one we tried proved to be the answer. So now we had some sense of what was going on with her heart. There was nothing that prevented our staying in Brazil. Our lives were invested there in training students for the ministry.

That medication enabled Doris to enjoy regular heartbeat for years afterward, with only very infrequent episodes of irregularity.

The normal pattern for missionary service was four years overseas followed by one year back in the States. That allowed the children to have a sense of being rooted in their two cultures, and enabled us to visit the churches that were underwriting our ministry financially. After two such terms I was invited to join the administration of the mission. We soon relocated to Cleveland, Ohio, that has been home for us since 1980. It also situated us in one of the finest centers of medical care in the nation. As Candidate Administrator, I oversaw all of the recruiting and orientation of new missionary personnel, including the 15-day Candidate Orientation Seminar each July, among other duties.

It took 18 years before we finally got to return to Brazil in 1997. That trip included some weeks back in Manaus with old friends, both Brazilian and American. Once we were back in that oppressive humid heat, Doris' heart began doing its funny dance again. An American missionary doctor was concerned enough that he telephoned our cardiologist in Ohio and they agreed on some other medication, and on the wisdom of her getting a pacemaker. By that time the devices were in common use and had a good track record for stabilizing heart rhythms.

Early in 1998 Doris had her first pacemaker installed at the famed Cleveland Clinic. Its threshold was 60 beats per minute, so her pulse would never be less than that. When her pulse was above 60 bpm it indicated that her heart was functioning well without the extra boost. The installation of that device included her constant need for "blood thinner" medications (really an anticoagulant rather than a thinner)(and not necessary for all pacemakers) and a also simple blood test every month or so. The testing would track her body's resistance to unwanted blood clots in the vascular system and help regulate the levels of clot-preventing medication. Those visits to Doris' own doctor simply became part of our regular routine, and we took it in stride. In the passing years the test itself became simpler and faster. The old PT test was a Prothrombin Time test to measure how quickly coagulation occurs in a single drop of blood. This was updated to the International Normalized Ratio, or INR, so a nurse now has results in a few minutes. Simple!

The miles of arteries and veins in our bodies include junctions and corners where blood clots can potentially form. If clots break loose rather than dissolve back into the blood they can clog a blood vessel. "Thrombosis" is not a rock band or new flavor of coffee, but a clogged pipe. If that should occur in a lung or in the brain it could have disastrous consequences.

Have you heard some people raving on the radio about the dangers of warfarin? They even call it "rat poison" to warn people away. That is grossly misleading and unfortunate. ANY medication can have side effects, especially if taken in megadoses. Many medications in common use, purchased over the counter, can have serious consequences if taken beyond dosages recommended in the package or by a physician. warfarin really is used as a key ingredient in rat poison, but only because it works so effectively, and in that odd application it is in massive doses that are fatal to little critters.

My mother was a research chemist in medical research. A key part of the fine tuning of therapeutic medications was the optimizing of dosages in micrograms of medicine per kilogram of body weight, tested and retested. They found the optimum dose for desired results, so medications are trustworthy as safe within prescribed limits. The goal is to enjoy the beneficial effects of the medication using the minimum dose possible. Coumadin (or generic warfarin) is safe, inexpensive, and proven over decades of use. Doris takes it every day in its carefully monitored dosages with no problems. Other anticoagulants have come onto the market that work well with their own side effects, limitations, and high prices.

Here in Medina, Ohio, southwest of Cleveland, we live within walking distance of our hospital, or a short drive to the doctor's office. The testing is very handy. Doris' brother Don also needed a pacemaker as they apparently inherited the same cardiac tendencies from their father, though in his case without rheumatic fever. Don did not have the same convenience for regular PTs so he did not want to take the anticoagulant. In time he was felled by a major stroke, followed by a second one while in the hospital, and did not survive the double blow. Doris was able to go see him during the three weeks that he was clearly failing, and both were thankful for their final conversations, until they meet again in Heaven.

The stakes are high. Our bodies were created with a variety of warning buzzers. But buzzers only warn. We heed the symptoms and take responsible action to maintain our health. Even proper diet and exercise do not guarantee our survival to advanced age. So Doris had the pacemaker installed, took the proper medicines, and did the regular testing to track important criteria affecting her health. That allowed her to relax and go about her normal frenetic pace of life and work. Into the 1990s she had worked for years as the office manager of our large church and its Christian school. She added to that much of the care for her aged mother who finally accepted our invitation to come live with us. Each of these was a full-time job. No wonder Doris got the license plate BZY LADY for her teal van!

Having taken all due precautions, we did not live under a cloud of worry about some thunderbolt out of the blue. Watch out! Some odd symptoms pointed Doris' doctor toward a colonoscopy. It was a routine matter (once you got past the yukky prep time) and that was done by a fine GI specialist in our hospital close to home. When the doctor called me aside for a report I kind of gulped. He had good pictures of a terrible reality. I stood there calmly conversing with him as if there were not a runaway freight train scrambling my brain at that moment. Despite the outward calm, inside my head I'm screaming, "Cancer? Whaddaya mean cancer? My Doris?!!"

I asked calmly, "Does Doris know?"

"I told her, but she might not remember."

But when I went to her she was fully aware of the doctor's quiet words engraved in her brain. The calm we displayed was really numbness. It bothers me when TV reporters show an accused murderer hearing the jury pronounce him guilty, and they say, "He showed no emotion at all. What a hard-hearted man." No, the internal tornadoes that many people experience don't show on the TV screen, but that is not the whole story, by any means. We feel a LOT more than we show.

For many people, including some in both of our families, the "C" word was a death sentence, but less and less so due to earlier detection, as in our cases, and improved treatments.

So our first major health adventure was quick surgery and mild rounds of chemotherapy. But that was our early quiz leading up to the major exam to come later on. It was only 1999. But you can see how the stage was set for the big drama to follow. Our health history is not simply a series of remote events. It is the accumulation of influences on our current health status, like the foundation that provides stability for a tall building. Part of our health history is what we inherited from our parents. We have seen how Doris and one of her two brothers continued the nature of heart problems experienced by their father. They could have been members of The Pacemaker Club that would be scattered around the country.

CHECK-UP: How has YOUR physical history contributed to the present state of your health? There are both favorable and unfavorable factors in your own life and in your primary blood relatives (grandparents, parents, and siblings).

2.

WHAT HAPPENED TO US?

Stage 2: What Happens in a Stroke?

One of Doris' many projects had been caring for a friend who got her own pacemaker at age 86. She then needed to move from her old third floor walkup apartment into an assisted living facility here in town. This move, and the downsizing after 35 years in one place, involved plenty of work but was a rewarding activity. It was not a source of stress or frustration. The friend's family got engaged in the process and deeply appreciated Doris' involvement.

Doris did some shopping for her friend and herself, grabbed a fast food lunch, and returned home. She set the bag of groceries on the kitchen table, turned and closed the door... and lightning struck! A blood clot inside her brain cut off the precious flow of oxygenated blood and that quadrant of gray matter instantly starved. She fell heavily into the corner of the wall and door, landing in a bent sitting position with her head skewed at an odd and uncomfortable angle, unable to move her left side. As she slipped in and out of awareness, she had no idea how to tell her body to even move, much less to get up. If she had worn a medical alert button then she would not have known how to use it. Something was drastically wrong!

In Doris' mind it seemed like 20 minutes went by before help arrived. Our daughter Margie lived in the attached apartment that was originally for her grandma, and she returned home from work with an alarming sense of urgency after getting no response to a call to her cell phone. In reconstructing the events from memory and evidence (like a friend who served Doris at Taco Bell) we found that Doris was on the floor for about two hours. Her thoughts ranged from bewildered prayer ("Father, what happened to me? Help me!), to ragged-edged terror ("What have I become?"), to a foggy sense of floating in a sea of nothingness.

For Margie, the nightmare of discovery began after she returned from a normal Saturday at work following her own ongoing recovery from surgery. She entered the door into her own apartment and came around the corner toward our kitchen and spotted a leg on the floor. In a millisecond of confusion she wondered why it was there. Another step forward and ... "That's Mom!" Margie's past years of experience as a nurses' aide caused her to recognize immediately a likely stroke. She lunged for the phone and called 911. Records show that the squad arrived in three minutes.

"Mom, What happened?"

"I don't know. I can't figure out how to get up."

Margie phoned a nurse friend who promptly drove to the house. She called in others in their circle of praying friends to support Margie as Doris was cared for and loaded into the ambulance. Doris promptly decorated its insides with her processed lunch. There is no glamour in patient care!

I was four hours away, conducting our mission's annual Candidate Seminar on the campus of Cedarville College. Back in "the olden days" before cell phones, people passed messages along. When a colleague came to tell me that I needed to telephone Margie at the Emergency Room of the Medina General Hospital I had only a sense of hollow dread.

"What happened??!"

"She would rather tell you herself." He exuded warm sympathy.

There was no softening the blow of the message that Doris had apparently suffered a major stroke. All my priorities changed in an instant. In the administrative team of the mission we were accustomed to cover for one another in times of need, and now it was our turn to receive help instead of give it. In record time I had handed off a list of responsibilities to colleagues, tossed minimal clothing into a suitcase, enjoyed the caring prayers of the gathered team, and hit the road homeward.

The guys were worried about my driving home alone, but I assured them that I was calm, not shattered or distracted beyond safe driving. During that trip I weighed the best-case and worst-case scenarios, and later told Dory I even cried. She was pleased, saying, "I need you to need me." It was a long, terrifying three hours home, even at those speeds.

I kept hanging on the word "apparent" describing a stroke, thinking it could well be something else. Or not. There were no good alternatives. Something was dreadfully wrong.

The Bible verse that kept coming to mind was "The Lord is in His holy temple. Let all the earth keep silence before Him." I not only sensed God's sovereign supervision of this whole matter, but knew that God knew what He was doing now, even if we did not. We would watch Him at work. That was true, but did not blow the terror away. The miles stretched on. The Seminar would continue on for nearly two more weeks, so for that time frame my work was covered. After that the situation would be negotiated.

It seemed an eternity for Doris as she lay paralyzed in Intensive Care surrounded by cryptic beeps and hisses, very much alone. Doctors and nurses were inserting needles and tubes, bustling her off to stuff her into gargantuan machines, and running test after test. Diagnosis must be accurate to allow appropriate treatment.

Somehow it never dawned on us to ask "WHY?!" or "Why ME?!" as if God owed us an explanation or an apology for allowing such an intrusion into our life together. The honest question would have been, "Why not?" Christians are a part of the human dilemma, part of the experiences of the race fallen from God's full favor, part of the suffering that falls to all people, not just to all other people. In that speeding car I remembered Job, the godly man whose suffering tested the reality of his trust in God and his closeness to God. Sure, he grumbled, and questioned, and failed the quiz, but he found that God passed the final exam.

Dashing directly to the ER Waiting Room at 10pm, I found Margie surrounded by her circle of close friends. Dr. Gary Anderson, the president of Baptist Mid-Missions, had gotten word from Seminar during my race home, and had come over immediately from his home. He was still a pastor at heart. Margie finally stopped for a good cry in her daddy's embrace. She had operated at her heroic pace to do all the right things and could finally pass the ball to Dad for a while. She knew I could not fix Mom, but knew I would take the helm and steady the ship of our family life. My own shakiness was not as apparent, but it was alive and well.

The human brain is a marvelously compact computer. Within that three-pound package are nearly one trillion complex cells that add up to 100,000 miles of wiring. Each such brain cell (*neuron*) has up to 1000 long nerve fibers (*axons*) with many connective hubs (*dendrites*). So the cells communicate with each other with flashes of electrical energy (*synapses*) or tiny bits of proteins and hormones. The "smart people" we all know don't necessarily have more brain cells, but they are known to be more deeply interconnected in their grids. If our little human brains are so complex, we can only imagine what the Creator's mind is like!

This gray sponge manages facts, imaginations, creativity, movements, languages, and emotions with incredible speed and ease. It even keeps churning while we sleep, both restoring its fatigued elements and categorizing the sounds that bombard us all night as "normal and safe" or "wake up and fix it!" Its ability to remember allows us to associate strange sounds we learned as children to still indicate the realities represented by those words. We only have to do first grade one time. Somehow it can receive and interpret the oral or written symbols (*words*) we use to communicate. It can take our elastic ideas and compress them into symbols (*words*) as our complex mechanism of vibrations and puffs shares concepts with other people. Our gray sponges can communicate with others' sponges through an incredible sequence of tiny technical exchanges from electronic flashes to mechanical compressions in air to vibrations of a membrane to a gadget that changes mechanical wiggles into electronic impulses (a transducer).

Our memory capacity is more than our home computers would need to download 25,000 HD movies. So why can't we remember where we parked the car or the name of that person right over there?

Our mind allows us to get beyond seeing just generic faces to recognizing real people and important stuff about them. In a crowd of thousands we can recognize a family member. It allows us to distinguish between important facts we need to remember and unimportant facts we can use and discard. Along with all these amazing abilities, the brain has plenty of redundancy, so parallel circuits can carry on the work done by other parts as needed.

But as a physical entity the brain is a convoluted blob of fat, mostly made of water and triglycerides. It thrives on the oxygen and nutrients that are delivered without fail by a network of arteries and capillaries within it. The "without fail" part only works when the oxygen supply does not fail. When the blood supply is cut off for even a few seconds some of those prodigious brain cells begin to die.

When a major artery is clogged the destruction quickly becomes catastrophic. Think of a stroke as cutting off some of the bridges and tunnels into New York City. Without those supply lines the city would be starved and paralyzed in a few days. The brain is much faster.

A little word like "stroke" does not begin to describe the disaster of a major "brain attack." The proper name for this catastrophic event is "a cerebrovascular accident," or CVA in medical shorthand. At least the word "stroke" does suggest the impact of something like the impact of a baseball bat on the brain within its protective case.

There are two main kinds of strokes, and neither one is good. The most common ones are **ischemic strokes** indicating the lack of oxygen supply. A blood clot (a *thrombus* of fat, calcium and cholesterol) can form in the carotid artery in the neck, or in other arteries within the head. Or, a blood clot (an *embolus*) can form in an artery elsewhere, or in the heart, and be swept into the brain where it can block off vital blood flow. Cells begin to die off, and the brain shuts down the body to prioritize its own protection. From the outside, we just see somebody faint and collapse.

A less common type is the **hemorrhagic stroke**. This can occur when an artery wall is weakened by uncontrolled high blood pressure, or at an abnormal spot that can swell outward like a balloon (an *aneurysm*) exerting unwelcome compression on neighboring areas of the brain. If the balloon bursts there is hemorrhage within the brain causing local compression and depriving other parts of needed nutrients. Some head injuries can cause these strokes.

Smoking, alcohol, and narcotics all conspire to weaken the arteries and contribute to the possibility of a major stroke. These common substances are not merely 'bad habits,' but are dangerous, contributing significantly along with other factors to future poor health.

A TIA, or Transient Ischemic Attack, may be a warning that conditions are ripe for a full intracranial earthquake. Even those temporary events must be regarded as serious despite quick recovery. In those cases when the clot dissolves quickly, allowing the blood supply soon to continue, the effects are temporary. What Doris experienced was no TIA, but was The Real Thing, without any hint or warning. It would not pass in 2 hours, or 24 hours, or 24 weeks, or even 24 months. The Monster had moved in to stay. Brain tissue had starved to death in seconds.

Immediate action is vital. This is not the time to "call the elders of the church to pray" (James 5:14). This is ambulance time! Pray on the run, and then at the hospital. Get help! First!

Remember the simple **STROKE ACRONYM** of symptoms:
- **F** ace   Does one side droop?
- **A** rms   Is one arm weak or numb?
- **S** peech   Is the person's speech slurred?
- **T** ime   Time is Critical. Call 911, fast!

CHECK-UP: What was the nature of the stroke, or other traumatic event, in your case? What were the symptoms, both before and after the event?

3.

WHAT DO WE DO FIRST?

Stage 3: In Intensive Care

Strokes can present strange symptoms: a sagging face, slurred speech, numbness of one arm or side of the face, or deep confusion that goes way beyond our normal "hardening of the smarteries." Sudden severe headache is a warning that something is amiss. Or there may be a major collapse, conscious or unconscious, as in Doris' case. Something is drastically wrong. Now what?

STEP 1: <u>Call the ambulance. Do not drive the patient to the hospital</u> since he or she is better kept calm in that home location. The EMTs may be able to begin treatment on the way to the hospital, or at least monitor vital signs and symptoms and send them ahead to the waiting medical team. This is no time for the "do-it-yourself" medical fumbling. Get professional help first. Do not stop to consult your favorite medical website. Call the ambulance. Dial 911 fast!

Take along the patient's wallet or purse so you have proper identification and insurance cards once the patient is taken inside. If you go to the hospital you normally use, much of your information will already be on file. Take the list of current medications. (Are they already posted on the side of the refrigerator to grab easily?)

Once you arrive at the hospital, the patient is whisked away into the inner sanctum of that temple of health. The family waits nervously, paces impatiently, seeks comfort as friends come to talk and pray. Everyone just wonders, "WHAT is going on in there??" We all feel helpless, wanting to DO something, hurting, hugging, waiting. It is time to remember that we have (probably) never done this before, while the physicians and nurses handle these cases every day. So while we stand by feeling like useless blobs, we are thankful for those who know what to do. And we are thankful for friends who come to the ER waiting room to attempt to lighten our load. It is time for just hugging and waiting together, sharing the uncertainty, consciously leaving the whole situation in God's hands, and waiting...waiting...waiting.

The doctors need to ascertain just what did happen, what kind of stroke it was, where in the brain the stroke occurred, how extensive was the damage, and how much of it is probably permanent. Not all of that will be known immediately. That calls for tests that can probe the inner workings of the brain, including EEG, MRI, CAT or PET scan or whatever is appropriate of the alphabet soup of medical mysteries. This is when details of the patient's medical history are vitally important, along with an accurate list of current medications.

In Doris' case, they could not do an MRI because that Magnetic Resonance Imaging technique involves strong magnetic fields that would literally rip her pacemaker out of her body. Other tests are available for that inside peek to map her brain in search of damage. They found plenty of destruction in the right frontal quadrant of her brain, the part that controlled the left side of her body. That was not the location of the main speech control center.

Doris had a CT scan which did not show any hemorrhaging in the first viewing, nor in a later thorough scouring of the details. The working theory that developed is that the stroke was caused by a blood clot dislodged from her left atrium due to a faulty mitral valve. She had long been a time bomb waiting to go off despite all our precautions. The fine neurologist on our case made it clear that this was not a passing matter, but was a major stroke that could be a life-changing event. She was preparing us for all sorts of potential bad news that even she could not yet define. Time would tell. This was a time when the phrase "God only knows" rang true.

Only a few days earlier Doris had undergone another colonoscopy as routine follow-up from her successful surgery for cancer three years before. The doctors had not transitioned in stages from one type of anticoagulant to another as was sometimes suitable for a surgical procedure. They said to just stop the Coumadin for three days and restart after the test. That was all it took to allow a blood clot to form, and then to be set free to eventually block a key artery to part of her brain. Most times that does not happen. This time it did.

We hear of "the magic bullet" that can be administered to stroke patients within a few hours of the stroke event, another reason to call the ambulance right away. In Doris' case, she was already using Coumadin so she would not benefit from any "clot-buster" that can help reverse the effects of the stroke for non-users of that drug. The doctors really do <u>need</u> to know what medicines are in use by patients.

Once the initial testing was done and Doris was stabilized, she was plugged into a stall in the Intensive Care Unit. ICU is a temporary setting for saving patients' lives and restoring their measurements to necessary survival levels. It is not a permanent location. A few family members were finally allowed to enter her room in the ICU. It is frightening to see someone you love hooked up to so many tubes and wires. It is also a relief.

You want to say everything and ask everything at once, but it is time to bring calm to the patient. This is no time for family members to dump their own emotions onto the patient. Friends and family who are deeply upset need to remain in the waiting room for a time. It does not help to ask, "How are you?" since the patient does not know either. For the time being, it is enough just to be there calmly.

Doris was conscious but subdued, able to whisper her appropriate and coherent comments. She was fully aware of her circumstances but did not have the emotional strength (yet) to face it all head on.

This was not just Doris' stroke; it was OUR stroke. This would clearly change both of our lives, but we could allow it to drive us together rather than come between us. Marriage is a three-way partnership when we understand that each of us is God's gift to the other, and He is the center and foundation of our lifelong marriage. The vows we made were not just to each other, but to God as we each accepted His gifts to us. That suggests that by giving us to each other He would also provide all of the resources needed to make the marriage successful. So there we were in ICU flitting back to the altar of the church starting it all off.

Doris does not readily adapt to changes, especially unexpected and unwelcome changes. But on that day she exuded peace. It was hard not to recall that her brother had died from such a stroke less than two years before. She was calm, partly from the trauma, vaguely aware that her whole left side was totally paralyzed, that her eyesight was somehow limited, and that life would never be the same. It is scary to have more questions than answers, especially when it seems that none of the possible answers are good for you.

The neurologist on our case sat with us so she could explain that this was "a major stroke," and not just a passing problem to be resolved quickly. This was clearly a life changing event.

I held Doris' hand and told her, "Nearly 40 years ago I promised to stand with you 'for better or for worse, in sickness or in health...' This is certainly that 'worse' part, but I am here to stay." She knew that, but I wanted her to hear that from me.

When tragedy befalls a woman, too many husbands just cut and run. Statistics show that about half of the men married to a woman who suffers a major disability will abandon her. They may claim that this would ruin their careers, or come up with some other rationale, but the reality is they are cowards who don't want to deal with hard responsibility. But a woman will normally stand by her man when times get tough. Good for them! Thank God for tough women. Somehow manliness seems to have overlooked responsibility.

The big surprise of the evening was when my brother Bob walked into our little room in ICU at 11pm that night. He was supposed to be in Wisconsin! It turns out that he as a pastor was taking a group of their church youth to Washington, D.C., and they were camping overnight at a church right in Medina. He had phoned our house to surprise us but found nobody home. We had telephoned his home earlier, but could just leave a message. His wife Linda connected the dots and by heroic efforts was able to rouse someone from the host church to go tell Bob that Doris was in the hospital just a mile away! It is hard to imagine such a scenario since in our day we would automatically reach for a cell phone to contact anyone anywhere.

Saturday night. Shadows hung over all of us at the end of that long, unthinkably difficult and dreary first day. Margie returned home and talked with our son Dave and family in Brazil to bring them up to date after her initial call earlier. Doris was sedated for sleep, medicated for a growing headache. I stayed in the "family sleep room" nearby ICU, hardly sleeping a wink. Hospitals are remarkably noisy, especially when your world has just exploded and you have more questions than answers. And especially when that sleeping closet is right next to the power doors that creak and thud all night long. We were all suffused with a sense of calm, but let's face it, we were numb with shock. Nothing could have prepared us for trauma of this magnitude.

Sunday morning came early, Day Two. Bob had already dropped in for a 6am visit mere minutes before I arose, and hit the road eastward with his team. Thanks for your surprise visit and loving support! The pace of activity in the hospital is reduced on Sunday with the weekend staff. Doris was awake and communicating better, though her headache was getting understandably worse. She had an inordinate desire for watermelon. She even joked that they did a brain scan and found nothing there, so her humor gene had not been crippled.

Sunday was not a happy day. That morning I had gone to church after a hospital visit and sat alone in a dim corner. One of the praise songs said in effect that when our days are at their worst, God was at His best. I resonated with that as one of the saddest days of my life unfolded so unpredictably. But I was comforted to know that God was in charge of the bad days and not just the good days. It is easy to praise the Lord when all is going well, and we can praise the Lord on a really lousy day as well. God is not brought down by our sorrows, though He accompanies us through our valleys of despair. He walked there too. Some complain, "If God is so good, why doesn't he stop our suffering?" He will, but in His own time and way.

Through the course of the day of testing and resting there was a stream of friends who dropped in for a brief visit with a flower, or a prayer, or an offer of help when the time comes. People came from our church, from Margie's church, and from the church that had hosted Bob's youth team, now praying for us. Doris welcomed each visit, but was visibly sagging in strength and attention. She has no memory of many of the people who popped in and chatted briefly with her. I kept a pile of notes and cards, and a thick notebook of emails pouring in. She read that many years later.

We watched with alarm as Doris declined in vigor through that second day. Her headache was more intense, and she just wanted to sleep. It seemed to us that nobody was actively pursuing her case as doctors handed off shifts and salvaged what was left of their weekends. Margie raised some questions about Doris' sinking conditions and insisted on more attention.

On Sunday afternoon I posted a message on our answering machine and faced the mountain of emails coming from all over the country. Others came from around the world as our mission family was sent a prayer alert. So I set up a bulk mailing and sent out an email in two large batches as an essential news bulletin. People throughout the family and our broader circle of friends and colleagues were aware.

As Margie and I debated which of us would stay in the "family sleep room" that second night, we watched an Amish grandpa from 50 miles away move in. We were glad to live within walking distance of "our" Medina General Hospital so somebody else could enjoy the benefits of the guest room.

Monday, Day Three, was a down day. Doris' brain swelling was the greatest danger. Only then did hospital folks explain that Doris really should not have so much stimulation. She should be allowed to coast with minimal brain activity. Please tell us! This is our first time through this maze of experiences. The key issue was the patient's needs, not just orderly protocol in the ICU. We could meet folks in the lobby, pass along information, and reduce traffic into ICU.

The event was now confirmed as a "massive stroke," not good news. One outside nurse suggested that we start planning a funeral, a totally inappropriate comment (that led to her not being called in to work there any more). Doris remained fully paralyzed on her left side, but was swallowing safely so she could be fed soft food. I reminded myself that if our roles had been reversed, Doris would not hesitate to feed me, and so her example encouraged me. Every bite was a simple "I love you" in motion. Her pain continued with her downward slide toward sleep and potential coma. It was a terrifying day, even with the moments of encouragement.

The neurologist on the case came back in Monday evening instead of her scheduled visit Tuesday morning for analysis. Margie also came in then and was alarmed that Mom had turned passive. She alerted the neurologist that yesterday she was talking freely and now is not responsive at all. The doctor reacted quickly to Doris' decline and shouted orders for a CT scan "stat!" She insisted that they begin the administration of strong medications to counteract the swelling in her brain. That most probably saved her life.

One medicine would reduce brain swelling but make her groggy. The other one would work on other factors and also increase her alertness. So the 'downer' was a constant drip feed and the 'upper' was given before mealtimes or examinations.

We had earlier phoned our son Dave who was working in Brazil with his family in missionary service, so he was aware of his mom's situation. I asked one of the doctors if she felt the family should be called in, and she pushed the desk phone over to me saying, "I would. Here, use the hospital phone." So they would be in the air from São Paulo to Cleveland within 12 hours with their three young children in tow.

Margie's prayer circle came by again to surround us with prayer and a group hug. The outpouring of such loving supportive care by so many was overwhelming. We were used to being on the giving side of the equation, so we knew the joy of such giving and let others have their day with us.

In my *Diary of a Stroke* I wrote that day,

> Perhaps I have been improperly calm about all this, but I have truly come nose to nose with the shocking reality of the prospect of the loss of my beloved wife of nearly 40 years. It is scary. Sure, many others pass through widowhood successfully, but I recognize all the more personally how profoundly I depend on Dory for the general dimensions of life

in our family. She is a gift from God, just the one I need. A week later she would ask me how it felt to face the loss of my wife, and I assured her it was an unnerving prospect.

The next two days finally allowed us to enjoy some improvement. Doris was not out of the woods in terms of life-threatening dangers, but the medicine to reduce swelling was working well. We at least felt like she had passed an important milestone. Nobody told us until a long time later that nobody expected Doris to survive the second night in ICU! Sometimes ignorance really IS bliss.

There was no need for her to rush into last-minute cramming for some heavenly final exam. The matter of Doris' salvation was settled years before when she trusted Christ to be her Savior. So we rest in His work rather than our works.

At one point I heard Doris whisper something that I did not catch. Try again? Say again? She was whispering, "Edwin Shaw!" That is the name of a fine rehab hospital near Akron, only a few miles away from home. Even in her extreme condition she was already taking charge of her recovery! I was amazed at the raw courage of this woman God had entrusted to me for life. No wonder she was such a steady rock of good sense and insight.

There were other reasons to rejoice. Family members were coming in, and we were careful to state that they came in support of recuperation, not to attend a funeral!

Our son Dave and family arrived at the airport at 9am of Day Five. Adam was 9, Ryan 6, and Shelly just 3-1/2. Hint: Do not bring little children into the ICU without prior orientation as to how that loved one will look and respond, or not. Actually, it is wise never to bring small children into an ICU because of all the microscopic monsters potentially floating around from all the other cases that need intensive care. That has become a rule at our hospital now.

Doris' big brother Bob and his wife Gerty drove over from Lombard Illinois. They shared tears in memory of Don's passing as well as for the present dangers. They kindly offered to stay in a nearby motel to simplify matters for everyone at the house.

Everything was rearranged at home for our family in from Brazil. I gave the family our whole upstairs so they could be together rather than scattered around with the boys in the basement bedroom. They needed the comfort of each other's company as well as we did. We blew up the "boingy bed" and had comfy places for all. It worked, In any case, I was always the first one up in the morning and the last one down at night, so it was fine for me to sleep on the couch. One of the dear older ladies at church was a West Virginian used to being up before the sun. So when she telephoned at 7:30am to check on progress as she prayed for us all, it was already afternoon for her, while it shattered our morning sleep.

One of Doris' cousins came over to help. Her goal was not to care for Doris in ICU, but to shepherd the grandchildren with fun activities while their folks concentrated on Doris' needs. That was considerate help that was a real relief for all involved. The kids also got to spend some days with their other grandparents close by.

During that week in ICU Doris came around in response to the medications that were pumped into her, and later CT scans defined the region of damage. To our surprise there were some basic therapy sessions despite her paralysis.

A speech therapist noted carefully how clearly Doris could speak, and tried to identify any flaws in how she articulated her thoughts. Were any elements of the speech mechanism affected by the stroke? She also paid attention to how well Doris could swallow liquids in her current state. It was wise to use a thickener in her liquids for a while to help her control her swallowing. That was not a single shot at analysis, but a daily visit to track and encourage progress. In a few days Doris was able to graduate off the thickener in liquids when she could safely swallow again.

I remembered reading that when people learn a second language after childhood that it is resident in a different part of the brain than our mother tongue. So I commented on something to Doris in Portuguese. She responded appropriately in Portuguese so we figured that corner of her brain was not damaged, wherever it was. A while later Doris commented to an ICU nurse that she had spoken to Bill in Portuguese. The nurse, having no context for such a bizarre statement, just smiled, "Oh, that's nice," probably ready to call a psychiatrist. I later explained why she would say such a thing since we had lived in Brazil for years.

Some medications can have fascinating side effects in a brain that has suffered an explosion. For a while, Doris was convinced that she had been picked up in a police sweep of a store parking lot along with all of the party girls in town. She would not be convinced that she was hallucinating. At least if she disappeared we would know where to look for her! She wondered how her doctor had even found her.

Every couple of days I was sending out an email update but found that the system would not take my mail. I called and found out they thought some spammer had taken over our account because of the volume and frequency of the emails. We got that straightened out, and I did not need to be protected from myself, so the mails went on. Now there are wonderful websites like CaringBridge for keeping up-to-date reports available and supportive messages coming in.

It became apparent that the immediate threat to life was past, and it was time to move out of ICU, a temporary, life-saving stage, to a regular hospital room for step-down observation. Then it would be time for a different sort of intensive care in Edwin Shaw Hospital. That speech therapist came to the room first thing in the mornings, singing a sweet little song she had written for her own daughter. It was a special touch. A social worker at the hospital guided us through the next transition with all the necessary paperwork, answering our many questions, and caring deeply about our struggles. Addled as we felt, we were grateful for the counsel of those who know the ways through the maze.

Dave and Val had reminded Mom that they came to encourage her along and not to attend her funeral. They would stay in the States long enough for her transition to the therapy hospital and then head home to Brazil. Doris was deeply grateful for their coming, for their encouragement in a tough time, and for the first time to see the grandchildren in a couple of years. In times of need there is nothing like supportive family – in short visits.

Still, that transition to therapy would prove to have complications of its own.

CHECK-UP: How was YOUR experience in ICU or first days?

4.

THERAPY? WHY BOTHER?

Stage 4: The in-hospital therapy

We were amazed, and somewhat bothered, that on the second day that Doris was in ICU some therapists from the hospital had her sitting up. They gently extended her arms to the front and side, insisting that she keep her eyes open to watch. They held her loosely to see if she could maintain her balance while sitting on the edge of the bed, which she could not. It seemed ludicrous to us when she had no control over the left half of her body. But therapists know the wisdom of starting right away to remind the patient's brain that it is responsible to control her balance and movements. They knew better than we did what limits guided the process. We knew enough not to complain that such early exercise was pointless and they should just allow her to rest.

One of the therapists lifted Doris' limp left arm and asked, "What is this?" When she answered, "My left arm" the therapist was relieved. Some person with strokes do not recognize their own bodies, but Doris could own that strangely detached arm as her own. That was good.

As we watched the professionals at work we were amazed and grateful for all they knew that we were previously unaware of in caring for patients. Margie had more patient care experience than I did, so she was able to orient us all as to what was going on and why. That helped us to cooperate instead of interfere with the normal procedures that go on in Intensive Care. They know what they are doing, and we just kept out of the way, even while insisting that one of us would always be there with Doris.

After about ten days in ICU and the step-down unit it was clear that Doris' cerebral swelling was under control, and that her vital signs were stable. One of the key rescue medications was no longer needed. She could eat safely when fed. They surely have other specific criteria related to the release of patients to move from the general hospital to the therapy hospital by ambulance.

It was heart wrenching for me to see my beloved wife strapped to a gurney in such a helpless state. I held back tears and wanted to yell, "Treat her gently!" (They already were.) I followed along to Edwin Shaw Hospital and found that the transfer went smoothly, a familiar operation for those who do all of that every day. This was a half hour from home, and was to be Doris' home for the next month or so. Home. That seemed so distant, so remote. Would she ever get home again? How could she cope, feeling utterly helpless? At that point I was more of a wreck than she was!

We were drained and it was just getting started. Doris was now in the hands of physiatrists (fizz-EYE-a-trists) who specialize in restoration of how the brain controls the body, especially the musculo-skeletal machinery that allows us to function well. **Physiatry**, or rehabilitation medicine, blossomed as a therapeutic field following World War II, and is now a multidisciplinary field in hospitals and rehab clinics. I had never even heard of such doctors, and now we were in a hospital full of them, along with the various kinds of therapists and their aides who did the daily hands-on therapeutic exercises.

The Shaw experience began with their thorough evaluation of Doris' history and present condition. That provided a realistic baseline from which to measure her improvement.

The days were structured with regular therapy sessions morning and afternoon. Rest was part of the therapy. Visiting hours were regulated since the patients were busily working on their recovery from all sorts of traumatic experiences. Some suffered brain injuries or strokes, and others were victims of falls, car crashes, or amputations. But the common thread of desire to recover created an aura of acceptance of one another and a sense of community support. The place hummed with optimism and the expectation of recovery – not always full recovery, but return to the highest degree of function that conditions allow. And part of the therapy is learning to accept new limitations.

We went into therapy planning to work toward full recovery. We knew that might not be our new reality, but we would work with that goal in view. If we had to accept limitations we would do so, but only after making every effort to get beyond them. This is when Doris' hard-headed Dutch realism was a source of strength. She never was a quitter, and she was not going to aim for less than full recovery. That meant lots of hard work, but she was no stranger to hard work. The work involved two main types of therapy, along with others.

PHYSICAL THERAPY (PT) deals with overall motor control of the body for balance and major activities like walking and moving the arms. The problem Doris had was not that her left leg and arm were weak or damaged. The problem was in the brain, the control center. The repeated motions of the body with conscious attention would, in time, remind the brain that it is responsible to direct those movements. So repetitious movements consciously driven by the patient facilitate the brain's remarkable ability to make new neural connections and take up control again. So therapy may appear to be dull repetition, but it is an elemental teaching process with a zillion little "aha!" moments firing off invisibly every day.

The brain gradually catches on and makes new connections to bypass the burned-out circuits. Some cannot be rewired, so there may be residual weakness. In Doris' case, her entire left side was affected by the stroke's damage to her right frontal lobe. Her brain had to be reminded by practice how to move her left leg so she could walk.

OCCUPATIONAL THERAPY (OT) deals with the finer work of the hands, or really, from the elbows on down. Such activities of daily living, called ADL, are the necessary linkage between our intent to act and our actions. Movements of both her hands had to be coordinated by the brain. The fingers have to relearn how to cooperate and how to function independently of each other. The first time around as infants, we had a year or two to accomplish all that. Now, as adults, we compress that into a month, at least to get started.

Exercises carefully teach hand-eye coordination as controlled by the brain. Every patient is different, and the therapists showed amazing patience with their patients to positively reinforce every minor effort and victory in very simple exercises. The improvement is in the brain, not in the hands, so mental attitude is vitally involved. Doris had two complicating factors that entered the equation.

At first she had lost left-side vision in both eyes, though that did return to normal within the first year, to the great surprise of some. She still did have the common tendency to neglect everything on her left side, even losing sight of the mashed potatoes on the left side of her dinner plate. She often wondered what time it was, not having noticed the wall clock on the left side of her hospital room. One of the OT exercises was to remove colored pegs from five rows in a device. But she had only noticed the two rightmost rows, ignoring the ones on the left side. That called for conscious attention. "Look to the left" was the new mantra.

Her other problem was that with the stroke she lost all feeling on the left side of her body, at least surface sensitivity. When people came near on her left side she would not be aware of them. Or someone who tapped her left shoulder got no attention. There is danger in not feeling pain (until it is deep pain of heat or cold or pressure) or even in not being aware of just where her left hand might be. Sometimes it floated, or ended up plopped in those mashed potatoes on the left side of her dinner plate! Then she could really feel the burn.

The process of therapy was both an agony of impatience and a litany of tiny victories, reinforcing the microscopic gains in control. We remember tearfully celebrating Doris' first step with her left foot on the parallel bars! Her leg was always fine, but her brain had to wake up to its responsibility to run the thing.

We remember the rush of victory when she first picked up a sheet of paper with her left hand! It takes an incredible degree of coordinated control for fingers and thumbs to conspire to do the same job gently. For robotics engineers that is a nightmare of gadgeteering. Normally our brains handle that seamlessly, but when we consciously have to make each part happen we marvel at the complexity with which our gray-matter computers have been created.

Then we learned that the control commands for letting go of that sheet of paper involve an entirely different set of muscles and circuits. Learning that release step was an entirely different new skill. Who knew?

On one quiet evening I was alone with Doris in her room at Shaw, after the aides had prepared her for bed. As we talked, the tragic nature of her stroke came home to her with its full weight. She had cried before, but this was the release of all the pent-up emotion after weeks of hospital days. It was a good cry, a soul-wrenching, pathetic, quiet, cleansing cry in the arms of her husband who felt it all just as deeply. She was not demanding anything from God or from me, but was facing her hard and tenuous future with total honesty, with grit and realism. She said she was crying for what she has lost and what she never had. This was profound and agonizing sobbing, a healthy cathartic cry, not the first and certainly not the last.

A friend of ours who had been paralyzed in years past wrote, "It is fine to cry; we need to cry; but we do not give ourselves over to crying as our lifestyle. God knows our hearts." I sat with her, deeply moved myself, feeling that I had never loved her more, even as a bundle of need and pain. It was not pity, but love that hurts because I knew I could only wait with her and welcome her relief in tears, since I could not fix this for her. Only God knew what was in store for us. But it was for US, not just for her. And it was FOR us, not against us.

So every day there were hours of PT and OT, with timely assessment of progress. Recreation and new friendships were a vital element of the healing atmosphere, along with meals and personal care by skilled aides. Doris found herself ministering to other ladies just by listening to their woes with a caring heart. Everyone added a piece to the puzzle as the big picture slowly came together. LIFE would go on! It would be different, but it was life, her life.

By this time I would go in to my office in the mornings and detour to Shaw Hospital in Akron for evening visiting hours. Life was going on.

Once it was clear that Doris was stable and improving, it was time for Dave and Val to return to their own life and ministries in Brazil. They had planned to stay through the transition into therapy and then hit the air homeward. After a couple of days at Edwin Shaw Doris had a spell of not feeling well, but part of that was anticipating missing the grandchildren. They said their tearful thank yous and good-byes, and I drove them up to the Cleveland airport to begin their southward journey home. Val's folks came to the airport as well to see them off. Just having family come for support in those vital weeks was worth the effort.

The run to the airport and back took a bit over two hours. Once back at Edwin Shaw Hospital I went right up to Doris' room. Her bed was empty! All her belongings were gone! Did I go to the wrong room? No. I knew she was feeling worse and worse, but not THAT bad. What happened??!! Where IS she?? (Me? Get excited? I did that time!)

The doctors had examined her, consulted with her primary care physician, and agreed that she had some internal gastric problems that called for a regular hospital. Doris had insisted on being taken back to Medina General Hospital just to be near family for our convenience. So on my dash back to Medina I actually stopped at a gas station to telephone [Doesn't that sound like something archaic out of the Dark Ages? OK, I was the technologically challenged one who had not yet gotten a cell phone!] Margie to assure her I was on my way and find out what was going on. What WAS going on??

Long story short, the medicine that worked so well to reduce swelling in the brain can also cause weakening of some tissue. It seems that the site of Doris' colon resection from cancer surgery three years earlier had gotten brittle and sprung a tiny leak. A gas leak can cause sepsis and quickly become a life-threatening situation. This was just a strange interruption in the already strange therapeutic process after a life-altering major stroke. Enough, already! So Doris was back in ICU for post-surgical follow-up, wondering if we needed season tickets at the hospital!

One evening, while Margie was getting Doris ready for bed as the short-staffed aides were all busy, she imitated what the nurses and therapists said daily. Taking her mom's limp left hand in her own she said, "Squeeze my hand, Doris." This time she DID! A full month after her stroke Doris made her first voluntary movement! It was just a slight movement of her fingers, an inch or so, but her brain told her left hand to squeeze, and it squoze! They squealed with joy and did it over and over again.

We were all goosebumps and praises to God. It was like the sunshine breaking through a wall of dark clouds. There was HOPE! This was the first of what would be many more tiny steps in response to weeks of patient therapy, showing the brain over and over and over what it can and must do. It really is paying attention. Doris was waking up!

Surely an important dimension of the healing process is the patient's own expectation of improvement. That comes about in response to therapy for body and mind, but also by the encouragement of friends and family. Knowing that the Lord is in charge of the process, using all of these factors, allows a trusting soul to rest confidently in that goodness of God. Such faith does not guarantee complete recovery, but does facilitate what improvement the conditions will allow. What a lift it was, to experience that one moment of significant progress!

It was time to get back to work in the routines of OT and PT. Due to the ongoing healing from the surgery, Doris' program focused more on work with her hands for a while. But there was new energy and anticipation. Each day some of the exercises were just a tad easier to accomplish, and she could move on to more complex work.

The calendar does not stop just because we have tragic situations. Our fortieth wedding anniversary came along while Doris was still in Edwin Shaw Hospital, but we had made no special plans. Margie had! To our surprise she came into the patients' dining area with a checkered tablecloth and a basket of BBQ ribs, flowers, and some cards and gifts. SHE was the real gift! So we sat at our own table for a private party as the folks sang their congratulations. My card for Doris included a bright coupon done in a computer template: "This coupon is good for all the loving care, patient therapy, support, prayer, and encouragement you will ever need from me." Below my signature flourish it continued, "(No expiration date) (No cash value) (Non-transferrable)."

Some dear friends of ours who had moved away from Medina had telephoned to see if they could visit Doris that day, not knowing it was a special day for us. Their timely visit made it all the more special. I told Doris someone was coming but would not say who it was. So Herb and Sondra were an uplifting surprise just when one was helpful.

The time came for another major move. Doris' incision was healing well so the surgeon gave her permission for a return to more rigorous therapy. Our checklist was amazing when compared to what she was like only six weeks earlier.

➤ She stood confidently in the parallel bars, controlling shifts in her weight and positions.
➤ She could take faltering steps in the parallel bars.
➤ She could move her left hand around the therapy table (supported in a sling) to perform simple tasks.
➤ She could lift her left arm a bit while reclined.
➤ She remembered to look leftward to enjoy that side of her little universe.
➤ She rubbed her affected arm with cloth or items of varying textures to awaken conscious sensations of feeling.
➤ She enjoyed general success in getting to the bathroom.
➤ She objectively discussed her future living conditions.
➤ She sought continuing spiritual development.
➤ She amazed people with her realism with emotion but not overwhelmed by self-pity or pervasive anger.
➤ She regained her natural smile, healthy color, and warmth.

This progress allowed a move to the Acute Care section for double the daily load of therapy. Improvements were coming along daily by then, and this extra work could accelerate the restoration of control. It was also time for Margie and me to attend a major assessment with the case manager and physiatrist to talk about prognosis. We also signed up for our training sessions for home exercises, transfers, equipment needed, refitting the house, and other such practical issues that naturally attend a return home. Doris' pacemaker never was a factor in this whole event. It assured us that even when other organs struggled, her heart beat quite regularly.

By now we could go out for a wheelchair walk around the hospital grounds and parks. It was early September, still pleasantly summery, just to talk, or cry, or pray, or practice some of her new moves like "kicking the soccer ball" with her left leg. Progress came in spurts followed by several days with no apparent improvement, just pausing to consolidate the gains into a growing repertoire of skills. Soon she was walking down the hall with a therapist, always with her gait belt around her for a constant grip. Part of this was getting accustomed to her new leg brace, from underfoot to just under the knee, as a permanent member of the family.

Margie was then working as a hair stylist, so she would wash and set her mom's hair once in a while. That gave a huge lift, and nice comments from fellow patients who wish they had the same. When a woman looks better she feels better. That provokes healing.

We got permission to go for a drive in our van if Doris would stay in the van. It allowed us to check out how our present van would work for her needs (just fine, thanks). It also allowed a good lesson in the transfer process as therapists walked me through the process of a secure move from wheelchair to van-with-seatbelt. No sweat! A simple drive around town and a stop for a favorite sandwich became a memorable treat after life in the desert.

Nine weeks after the stroke I was able to take Doris to a hot air balloon festival with 25 balloons in various stages of inflation and eruption. We talked our way right onto the field between a couple of teams. Once the gas burners were fired up the incredible globules of bright colored designs came to life before our eyes and lurched into the air. Doris had always wanted a balloon ride, so this is as close as she would get, and it was total delight. Her spirit was soaring with the balloons and their riot of colors!

Life would never be the same. I was grappling with the changes due in my life as well as Doris', and knew I needed resources. Friends came to mind: one who had cared for his wife through more than 20 years of her MS with increasing demands, and also another friend in the same situation who had not stayed around to help. What a difference! A doctor friend had carried his wife in and out of church services with her vacant stare and non-communicativeness for years on end. Maybe she appreciated the interaction; maybe not.

I got the little gift book **A Promise Kept** by a former college president who stepped down to care for his wife as she sank deeply into Alzheimer's Disease. He remarked, "I don't *have* to care for her, I *get* to care for her." He noted that as she had tended to his needs for 40 years, if he tended to hers for 40 years he would still be in her debt. Another friend, a shirt-tail relative, had cared for his wife tenderly through her three-year struggle with cancer and was lovingly with her at the end of her journey. So there were models before me as to how to go about this new life successfully (or not).

A therapy hospital is NOT a vacation spa. It is a workplace. The normal post-stroke treatment span is about one month, though each case has its own dimensions. The focus is on ADLs, those common activities for daily living, to facilitate adjustment to self-care or others' care at home rather than in an institution. The aim is full life at home.

As Doris improved she walked the hall, climbed the stairs, and amazed the OT therapist with her new dexterity. Doris ended up with 44 days at Shaw, in part because of the interruption for surgery. But the key criterion is continuing progress and improvement. The purpose of the hospital is not long-term care-giving. There are many such care facilities in most communities for those who need extended therapy. We scheduled out-patient therapy in a facility much closer to home, having also considered a transition stay in a nursing home near to home, but Doris was ready to go home, to her own home, her own bed, her own bathroom, and her own dealing with her new limitations that made her world shrink.

Yes, there IS a larger world out there. Patients go through a range of emotions in a resident therapy center. They may arrive numb with shock, relieved that there is care available. Hope rises, but sinks when they realize how much of the success of the project depends on their own determination to improve and to work hard to recuperate. Then they get tired of the newness of it all, having someone feed or bathe them, dreading the bedpan, complaining about the meals (however good they may be), and being surrounded by people worse off than they are. They don't want to stay, but don't want to return home. As they improve they realize that the therapy really is helping and the therapists and doctors really do know what they are doing. In time, they actually look forward to returning home. Home! Aaaahhh!

The therapy is to impel the patient toward recuperation. That is the obvious part. The less tangible part is the training of family members for continuing therapy at appropriate levels at home. That is not the technical training for which therapists are licensed, but protective and prudent oversight of gentle exercises that the patient is to continue on his or her own. The family provides a positive atmosphere of kind acceptance and encouragement to motivate ongoing improvement. We also learn not to do more than is needed so the patient grows in independent living.

The time at the therapy hospital or other rehabilitation center is also a time of adjustment for the spouse and family of the patient. Their lives will also change in more subtle ways. These weeks allow rethinking of how life at home will adjust and continue. The patient will learn to respect the autonomy and needs of the caregivers.

We do not get to bring along the army of helpful therapists and aides who have made our lives so much more enjoyable in the hospital. They are the invisible helpers who worked long hours when family members were not there. They helped with meals, personal hygiene, bathing, dressing, and other ADLs, careful to let – or make – the patient do as much as possible for herself in increasing measure. Once at home, we will be on our own for the next phase of recovery.

A stroke does not happen to one person. It happens to a family.
- If there are elderly parents still around, they wonder who will care for them.
- Children feel helpless when their personal Wonder Woman is clearly as weak as they are.
- The spouse of the patient feels tossed around as if caught in a clothes dryer.
- It happens to the faith community or social community which will rise up to support and encourage the family.
- The stroke affects the close friends who will occasionally help with visits, transportation, meals, cleaning, and other supportive tasks.

We are all in this together. How will it be different once back at home, feeling unfamiliar in a familiar setting?

CHECK-UP: What are YOU learning in your experience of a rehabilitation center that will be most helpful at home?

5.

A NEW FAMILY LIFESTYLE

Stage 5: Coming Home to Changes

When therapy began, the prospect of returning home was a source of terror. Doris ran through the catalog of daily household duties in her mind, checking off the ones she was no longer capable of handling. There was no comfort in a crazy notion like, "No problem! Bill will step up and handle all of those things and keep it all running smoothly." That wasn't even funny. I was not famous for operating the household smoothly, but could get too cozy with dust, and was deeply skilled at procrastination. For Doris, the naturally organized administrator, being even partially paralyzed was a nightmare! Life was one big question mark.

Margie and I went through the house to see what had to be modified to allow Doris to move about with her walker or wheelchair. Long before our own needs arose, we had sought a house with the ground floor all on one level. Flat floors were suddenly rare, an exception to architectural trends with a fashionable step-down dining room or other parts.

Our whole reason for moving to Medina had been to accommodate Doris' mother who was already using a walker and would probably need a wheelchair in her years with us. So in our initial remodeling of our "new" house we built a wheelchair ramp inside the garage and installed the higher geriatric toilets. That was in place. Hoodathunkit that it was really for our own use!

It was too early to consider remodeling the kitchen with lower counters for wheelchair access since we had no idea how much Doris would be able to keep doing. But around the main floor of the house we removed some excess furniture and all throw rugs. We measured doorways for wheelchair clearance. We located places where grab bars might be installed if needed to facilitate walking.

For the time being, we set up a bedroom area for Doris at one end of the living room. In time she could tackle the stairs, as she was already practicing in therapy. We installed a second railing on the up and down stairs so she would have grips on both sides. That would make a huge difference of access. But her PT lab had three steps up and down while the house had thirteen steps up to the bedrooms or down to the basement laundry and her sewing room. Sewing?

> Would she ever sew again? She had just begun quilting, so how could that continue? Will her fingers be able to manipulate the small pieces and the tools? Will her mind allow her to keep a zillion pieces in order? Only time will tell.
> Could she walk?
> Could she prepare meals?
> Could she drive?

Questions abound, and for an agonizingly long time the only answer is, "Wait and see how much agility and strength she recovers." The matter is further complicated in cases when the stroke has affected the speech or clarity of mind of the patient.

> Should we install a lift chair to get upstairs? Wait and see. Ok, ok.

One of the measures of success we observed at the therapy hospital was that Doris began making plans to make things work at home. She moved from dreading the return to a softer prison to a longing to be back in her own home. This was a major victory. She was very thankful that her saintly mother was already safely Home and not suffering by seeing her with this new condition.

Part of that victory was that both Margie and I were eager to have her home. Margie had worked in a nursing home as an aide during summers of her high school and college years, so her experience in patient care was very reassuring. When I was a teenager my one grandmother had lived with us for her final years. So the prospect of being caregivers was not totally strange to us. We described the gentle changes we had made at home for Doris. We assured her that we would do for her what she could not do for herself, but push her to do as much for herself as was possible. That sounded good to her too.

Doris wanted to be as independent as possible and was surprisingly adventurous as to how household routines could be modified to fit her abilities. All this was complicated, of course, by not knowing how far she would improve, once the rush of recovery was underway at an accelerated pace. It began with a slight squeeze, but that simply opened the door for a reawakening, a reconnecting. Doris' brain seemed to be enjoying a sense of, "Oh, I get it; I'm now supposed to <u>drive</u> this vehicle! I can't just ride along."

When a stroke patient is improving, consistent therapy can maintain a pattern of new rehabilitation through the next four to six months. Most of what a patient is going to recover will happen in the first quarter year and half year, tapering off after that through the first two years. Continuing growth far into the future is more in the area of developing new coping skills and just getting used to limitations. We find new ways to manage the difficulties that will always remain.

In our case, the time from Doris being whisked from home in an ambulance until she returned home in our van was ten full weeks, Saturday to Monday, including 44 long adventuresome days in Edwin Shaw Hospital. She was walking with a quadcane (as one of us gently held her gait belt), enjoying continence control, using her left hand in very limited ways, and remembering to check the left side of her universe. She was HOME!

We walked in to find a "Welcome Home, Doris!" sign near some fresh flowers cut from a friend's garden, and a party tray for handy lunches for a while. Once she was home it was easier for friends to drop in for a quick visit. People were thoughtful to keep visits short out of respect for her limited energy.

We enjoyed our own birthday party for Shelly, now back home in Brazil as she turned four years old. The birthday cake had its four candles and bright colors. So we got Doris some toys that would be helpful in therapy: a big soft ball for rotating her left leg with her foot on the ball, a set of alphabet blocks for stacking, and a bedside monitor to call me for nighttime help if needed, or Margie when I needed to be on the road. We were careful to call that a "patient monitor" rather than a "baby monitor." A friend dropped in for a very welcome massage for Doris' neck and shoulders. Nice party! I got in line, to no avail.

Within the first week at home we went to the therapy facility related to Shaw Hospital but only 10 miles away instead of 30. The careful evaluation concluded, "Well, you have a lot of work to do, but you have a lot to work with." Encouraging. We would begin with OT and PT sessions on Tuesdays, Wednesdays, and Fridays. I always traveled with a good book or two, or worked at my laptop "office." Doris found some new pains, but they were good signs of improvement as her body continued to wake up from its traumatized sleep mode. We also did milder exercise routines at home. She was one determined lady, still working hard at getting back her freedom to move. The grillwork on our stairway handrail at home was a great place for attaching therabands and pulleys for her workouts.

Doris' first Sunday back in church brought a flood of hugs and warm thoughts from many friends. After dinner at home from church friends we rested and then read together. We tackled that warm little book, **A Promise Kept**, and both cried as we enjoyed the love story of a caregiver and his wife who faced tragedy together. That lady's problem was Alzheimer's Disease rather than a stroke, but the husband's patient care for her was a love story in itself, a model I valued. I needed to drink deeply of such a spirit of self-giving.

A friend from church arrived with a heartening surprise. She brought some supplies and announced that she would be coming every week or two to clean house for Doris for the rest of that year. This was her gift to Doris and an offering to God of service that left us praising the Lord for her. Very thoughtful. After that we made other such arrangements, but her loving initiative was unforgettable.

One problem is always humming in the background. When someone has lost a quarter of her brain capacity, will that not affect functions of thinking as well as moving? While Doris did not undergo any major changes of personality, there were signs of deficits in several areas of her life. Her sense of smell was diminished. Her ear for music was distorted so it was harder to sing in tune without drifting into another key. Making decisions became a challenge, even in familiar issues. Short-term memory was more problematic than her long-term memory, sometimes a frustrating new reality.

At one point when she lamented, "My brain just doesn't work any more," I stated, "Look at it this way. Your hard drive is intact, but you have less RAM for processing ideas." That made perfect sense to an executive secretary who had lived on the computer for years.

In some stroke patients the speech control center is affected, or they cannot read any more. They know those squiggles represent sounds, but cannot make any more sense of them than we can of Chinese characters. Families will learn to adjust.

There are cases where very proper persons begin using really salty language. Somewhere in the brain we have all tucked away a file of 'words we know but never use.' If the normal 'dictionary' is damaged, those forbidden words may be the primary vocabulary the patient has. This is a time for understanding, not for judgmental indignation. Reduce the stress by comprehending what they are going through.

A wheelchair is both a liberating vehicle and a portable prison. The glory of the stroke has faded. The heroism has evaporated. Those supportive friends have been doing what they could, but they won't be as active for the long haul. What is starkly in your face is the prospect of some permanent deficit, the grief of loss, the remaining hard work of therapy, and the gradual nature of ongoing progress. It just isn't any fun. But this is a process of building hope.

Let's think about a basic **CHECKLIST for house and household.** These are not "jobs to be completed before Mom can come home" kinds of tasks. These are issues to be confronted and analyzed honestly in the family setting, some to be discussed frankly, some to mark modifications in duties and/or physical conditions. Give priority to the independence and dignity of the patient. Let her, or him, be an appropriate part of discussions.

1. **MOVEMENT** about the house. Is there room for a wheelchair? It may be a full-time or part-time location, but if a wheelchair is used at all there must be a way for it to get around.
2. **OBSTACLES** to free or safe movement. Are there small rugs or unnecessary clutter? Some items can be discussed with the patient so she participates in re-feathering her nest rather than coming home to a strange place. Many details can await the arrival of the patient at home to help decide them. It is her home too.
3. **SLEEPING SPACE.** Can the patient get to bed, and to the bathroom? Is a temporary bedroom facility helpful if it gives independence? Will a portable potty chair be

helpful at night? Will privacy be a problem? How does the change of space affect the rest of the family? How will clothing and other personal effects be available?

4. **BATHING** is essential to one's sense of dignity. How will she/he bathe? Will help be necessary? (Probably)

5. **MEAL PREPARATION** is best left to others during the first weeks at home. Friends may be willing to bring meals for a while, or even come over to prepare a meal in your kitchen. Much depends on the patient's emotional state as well as physical condition. Lift that load for a month for settling in. Someone else in the family becomes the resident chef, whether temporarily, or permanently. You can work out who decides on meals and shopping lists. Each family has its own kitchen culture and can negotiate what is best in the long run.

6. **KITCHEN MODIFICATION** depends entirely on whether the patient will return to preparing the meals. Some cannot for a while, while others never will be able to do that. Some never did, so little changes. The remodeling of the kitchen to accommodate a wheelchair should not be undertaken until it is deemed necessary and helpful. Don't decide all in advance.

7. **CLEANING HOUSE** is a bigger issue for women patients than for men (who can't see dust anyway). Find someone she enjoys and trusts to hire for a half day of thorough cleaning every other week or so. Let her oversee that part.

8. **HOUSEHOLD FINANCES** and similar matters have to be kept up to date. If the stricken person was the primary manager of the checkbook then it is time for the spouse to step up and learn the ropes.

9. **SPECIAL EQUIPMENT** will be added as needed: grab bars in the bathroom and shower, a shower seat, a "bed cane" on both sides of the bed to hold onto for help getting in and out (or a rented hospital bed for a few months), perhaps eating utensils with large handles, and a bib or apron. It is better for the patient to depend less and less on special equipment and function on his

or her own. But some is needed, especially at first. We're glad for local medical supply stores that have an amazing variety of geriatric equipment to make life simpler, and friendly folks who understand.

10. **TRANSPORTATION** is more of a problem if the patient is unable or unwilling to drive. So the caregiver becomes the chauffeur among many other new jobs. It consumes time, so take along a good book to read. Friends will be glad to occasionally take her shopping or for a doctor or hair dresser appointment. They need to be aware of any special needs and how to care for them. They must be able to assist in transfer in and out of a vehicle when a wheelchair is used.

Residual weakness is not some fault of the patient as if she did not try hard enough or could have done better. The development of new neural pathways may be blocked by scar tissue or otherwise hindered. Dead tissue is just that: dead tissue. There are fancy medical terms but the fact is that some damaged parts of the brain are beyond repair and cannot be replaced. Some functions may never return, or may partially return. Every case of stroke is individualized, varying with the location and severity of damage.

Doris will always have 'left-sided hemiparesis' which says her affected side is the vertical half ("hemi") of her body, to the left side of her midline. There she is weakened rather than paralyzed. The weakened condition is not in her arm or leg or skin, but in the controlling connections from the brain.

If she had doubled her efforts at PT and OT she could not have doubled the benefit of the therapy. Stroke patients are never to be blamed for not working hard enough, as if it were their fault. This is how she would be for the rest of her life, still granting gentle improvements both in dexterity and in managing her limitations of strength and movement. Accept it. Make the most of a new condition.

Three months after Stroke Day we did another inventory of Doris' current situation in October of 2002.

➢ She continues out-patient and home therapy with a positive attitude about minor improvements.

➢ She has occasional sessions of deep grief, with healthy crying and understanding support from the family.

➢ She functions independently in the bathroom, including bathing, limited mostly by reach and energy.

➢ She works around the kitchen from her wheelchair, setting and clearing the table, managing the dishwasher, planning meals with us. Friends were still bringing meals, but we asked to reduce to two days a week since we were overwhelmed with leftovers and the kindness of families in our churches.

➢ She dresses independently for the top half, and needs help with compression hose and tying shoes, etc.

➢ She can stand and walk when accompanied, using the walker or quadcane, but is still not steady enough to go it alone. She remembers the "nose over toes" mantra to help stand up, and does better at sitting down in a controlled manner.

➢ Her left hand is not integrated into normal body activity unless she gives it conscious direction, sometimes out loud. She can touch her thumb to any finger, and sometimes feel it, though release of a grip is still a separate function demanding concentration.

➢ She needs to give full attention to her walking when she moves about, so that is not a time for conversation. Let her do one thing at a time at her own pace.

➢ She sleeps more than before, often 11 or 12 hours, seldom calling for help in the night.

➢ She is grateful in spirit: to God for preserving her life, to Margie for her loving support and plenty of competent physical care, to her husband who has surprised her with his degree of patience and caregiving, and to many friends who express support.

We would work at home therapy, and go for out-patient professional therapy, but by the end of 2002 we had to accept the reality of how she was going to remain. Doris was not going to wake up from a nightmare and discover that none of this really happened. We could not rewind the tape and edit out the terrible stuff. God was not going to reach down from Heaven and say, "I was just kidding; be well."

This was not a surprise. We knew from the beginning that there could well be permanent limitations affecting her from now on, despite working toward complete recovery. I as her loving husband had to be sure that I accepted that reality, because a package of new responsibilities was rushing my way. How can I be a caregiver? I'm the wrong guy for this job! Help!

CHECK-UP: What adjustments to your physical circumstances at home, or other long-range facility, have you found helpful?

6.

HOW CAN WE HANDLE THIS?

Stage 6: Caregivers Step Up

The family is the God-ordained building block of society. Not all families function according to plan, but many do. When one part of the body is disabled, the other parts modify their functions to compensate for the lack. When one goes blind, the hearing gets more acute, or at least gets better attention to enhance awareness.

A vital part of the work of the therapy hospital is to train caregivers. The time in the hospital allows analysis of the special needs of the patient, the configuration of the dwelling, and the reallocation of the normal duties of running the house. Who will do what? An initial plan is formulated even though things probably rarely turn out that way. At least there is a plan to modify in terms of the new reality.

Some years ago a friend of mine suffered an unspeakable tragedy that left him a quadraplegic, paralyzed for life. His wife was wearing herself out being his arms and legs. What could I say to her from my own ragged experience? Thoughts tumbled out and eventually came together in a simple booklet. I gave that to the caregiver/wife and they read it together, finding it helpful, so it is abbreviated here. Change channels for this chapter to think as the caregiver rather than as the patient. In any case, it is a cooperative effort.

"Ten Commandments for Caregivers"

Instead of writing the "he or she" bit, I'll mostly speak of "she" as the suffering wife and "he" as the caregiving husband. This is my experience, and it is more unusual than the other way around. Please read this according to your own circumstances and do whatever switcheroo is helpful. We recognize the normal roles of the wife caring for the family (whether or not working outside) while the husband normally works outside and gets cared for at home. So we mere men are less equipped to deal with serious changes in the routines that are 'normal' at home. These ten suggestions are not listed in order of priority. They are all important. Try them on. Here are the first five guidelines.

1. THANK GOD FOR THE DISABILITY.

You need not be thankful that your beloved spouse or child or parent suffered some traumatic event that left her disabled. It may have been an automobile crash, a stroke, a major heart attack, an assault, a fall, the result of disease, the aftermath of less-than-successful surgery, or a zillion other debilitating events. Her life is now changed forever, and not for the better. Your life changed too.

You are not thankful that it happened, but you can thank God for the positive things that do come out of it all.

- ➤ This did not happen "back in the good old days" when she would probably not have even survived the ordeal, or would have suffered more primitive therapies and less effective medications.
- ➤ This will make you more sensitive to others who suffer, and able to be supportive to those in similar circumstances like you never could before.
- ➤ Friends have come out of the woodwork offering help of many sorts.
- ➤ You have peace that God knows what he is doing, even when you do not. This new condition is a gift from God, even though you never wanted it.

A thankful heart recognizes that God is in charge of the mess we find ourselves wrapped in now. We feel lost in a huge maze. But from his vantage point Father can see the way out. For the time being, all we know is that God knows what's happening, and why in his own economy. We are thankful for that.

The one who is disabled may find that her spiritual sensitivities have been heightened. Our spiritual makeup tends to compensate for the reduction of physical ability by increased interest in spiritual uplift and refreshment. One who cannot run can still pray, and will come to find intimacy with God a wonderful reality. Meanwhile, encourage spiritual vitality without getting preachy. Read together; pray together.

2. OFFER ONLY HOPE AND SECURITY.

When we married, we promised to be faithful "for better or for worse, in sickness and in health," and those down sides have come upon you. Remind her that your promise still stands. Remind yourself, if you need to, that you made a vow before God to care for her as long as you both live. Make it clear that this problem has come to both of you, not just her, and that you are ready to go with her through whatever it takes to survive and go on living.

Embrace the trauma as your own as an expression of love for her. She will not be abandoned to suffer through this alone, and needs to hear you say that lovingly. She needs to see you live that dedication to your mutual vows in order to enjoy the security of your loving care. She will be all the more dependent and needs to know of your willingness and eagerness to help her, just as she would have helped you if the tables were turned.

In this new economy there is NO place for sarcastic remarks, belittling comments, blame, or even the suggestion that she is lazy or incompetent. She would love nothing more than to be restored to full functions and go back to working circles around you. She cannot just 'snap out of it' and return to the old normal. Your supportiveness and sympathy are a vitally important lifeline. Be positive without being patronizing. Continue to speak to her or him as your beloved spouse, not as your patient.

Try to bring serenity into the sickroom. There is already an abundance of anxiety, so you do not want to feed that with more of your own. You may find it helpful to find an understanding friend with a listening ear and consolation for your own tears and fears. This is not a call for saccharine sweetness with your spouse, but for the time being you cannot unload more worries for which she may not have the emotional fortitude.

There is no way the caregiver can blame the fallen spouse for whatever was suffered. This is something that has befallen both of you together, not something that one did to the other. The caregiver never has ground to say, "Look at how you have ruined my life!" That is untrue, unfair, unjust, unloving. You may get angry at your circumstances, but you can never take that out on the one who has been traumatized. Keep that to yourself. Stay on the same side to support one another and let the tragedy draw you closer in mutual dependence rather than flip the magnets so they repel each other. You are not angry at her so much as frustrated with your new circumstances.

Your spouse must know that she can call for your help at any time she needs it. ANY time. You may negotiate what is a <u>need</u> and what is a <u>whim</u>, but in the time of need she can call without any embarrassment or hesitation because you are there for her. For some matters she can wait for your convenience, just as anyone needs to be considerate of others around her, but as a rule she will find you happy to respond with good cheer and consideration. There is no place in your new lives for an impatient, "Oh what do you want this time?!" That creates fear just when you want to project security.

3. AVOID THE 'OH, POOR ME' COMPLEX.

We quite naturally ask, "Why me, God?" and expect some sort of answer. We are really gently demanding that God be accountable to us and explain why hard things have happened to us. When phrased that way, we quickly recognize that it is not a reasonable demand. We can seek lessons, and think about some rationale, but do not want to find ourselves deep in self-pity and blaming it on God. The simple fact is that the human condition is less than ideal, and that some of the normal rain falls on our heads.

Here's a syllogism to try on for size: Some people get sick. We are people. Therefore, some of us will probably have a turn to get sick. That is reality, but is not much comfort. Remember that even if God did sit you down and explain all that he intends to accomplish in you because of this suffering, you still would not enjoy it (or it wouldn't be suffering). Maybe God does have some special reason for your hardship, maybe not. Ask, but don't demand, for grace to learn whatever He has to teach. This in itself will help us move beyond the "oh, poor me" stage, whether we are the sick one or the caregiver. Both are subject to such thinking. You can always find others in worse condition than you are.

You cannot blame yourself for the stroke, any more than you can blame her. Forget the tendency to accuse yourself, "I did terrible thing XYZ, and now she is suffering for it." Nonsense! There are medical reasons why people have strokes, and you are to be part of the solution, not of compounding the problem. Regret is normal. You wish this had never happened. But guilt is not applicable here. They may feel the same, but regret and guilt are vastly different.

4. ACCEPT HELP THAT IS OFFERED AND NEEDED.

Imagine for a moment that it was your neighbors who suffered what happened to you. Would you not be ready and eager to help them? Would you look down on them for needing help? Would you be willing to sacrifice a bit of your time to help with some tasks that have become difficult for them? Would you count helping your friends as a way of serving the Lord?

Now switch roles. It is <u>their</u> neighbor that has a need (that is, you). Can you not imagine that your neighbors (including families at your church) would have just as good an attitude toward you as you would have toward them? Even though you are accustomed to give help rather than get help, now is your turn to receive. Allow your friends to serve by doing some tasks which are a real help to you. Set aside the subtle pride that wants to go it alone.

You now have to live two lives: your own (somewhat reduced in scope) and hers (very reduced in scope). Do the math: 80% of your life duties + 50% of your spouse's life duties = exhaustion at 130%. You do need help. People will gladly bring in meals – for a while, a month or so, not forever. People will care for her so you can go to work – for a while, not forever. People will clean your house and mow your lawn – for a while, not forever. During that adjustment time when you are still dealing with trauma, feel free to accept the offered help without shame or pride. You would gladly help them; so allow them gladly to help you.

In time, you will find your own solutions to the new "normal" of your lifestyles. But that takes a while and those friends will gladly be true friends if you let them.

5. BE A LARGER PART OF HER WORLD.

Your spouse's world just shrunk down to a pinpoint. She will need more of your time just to be there, just to listen to her thoughts, just to be her eyes, just to share her lifepain with someone who really cares. If it is difficult to just get out of the house she will hesitate to "bother" you with another job or another trip or another favor. That draws her world in tighter.

She needs you more than ever. Be there!

A lot of the time now needed is just to be with her since she is limited in getting out to be with other people. You cannot be chained to the bedside, but must expect to just spend more time with her in the normal course of things. Some of your jobs can be transported so you can work while you are together, and many cannot. Some of "your" agenda will get postponed, some reduced, some dropped. This is a permanent change for both of you. Get used to it.

You will become a larger part of her life in general. A lot of that is due to her reduced mobility and jobs she simply can no longer do. If she cannot make her bed or reach heavy things on the top shelf or tie her shoes, those become your jobs now. More time on her agenda means less time on your agenda, and adjustments need to be made. You will go through cycles of trying this or that alternative, but you just don't get extra hours in the day or energy to do the work of two. You come to anticipate what she needs and provide that as part of your new lifestyle. Look for new things to do together which you both enjoy, and things you can do separately together. Bring joy into her life by your presence and attitude.

Your marriage has not ended just because of major trauma and limitations. Your friends are still your friends so you want to get out and around as much as your circumstances permit. Warm fellowship at church or elsewhere, and some normal exchanges with friends about things other than the key problem have a healing influence. Encourage such contact, and outside your own home or sickroom if possible.

CHECK-UP: Who are the primary caregivers in YOUR case? What help will they need?

7.

MORE ABOUT CAREGIVING

Let's finish up our *"Ten Commandments for Caregivers"* as we keep in mind that these are guidelines rather than laws to keep. Every family will adapt general principles to their circumstances. Until now we have focused on helping the patient, and now we look at helping her become more independent.

6. LET THE DISABLED ONE USE ALL HER ABILITIES.

There is another side to doing more for those with permanent handicaps. It is good for them to do as much for themselves as they are capable of doing. It is good practice. It is good for morale. It is good therapy. It fosters independence. It is good for you.

But there are new limits. There are some jobs she will never be able to do again. She grieves over that and needs affirmation that it is not by some fault, or laziness, or neglect. This is never a time for resentment on your part over being given jobs you never wanted. She never wanted this either, and it is new for you both. Live with it. As head of your home you are responsible to create an environment of support and love and harmony. Accept the adversity as from God, not from the devil, not from your wife. And while you're at it, do not blame God for the trouble, but thank Him for the help that comes along with it. We come to live a new definition of maturity.

Some tasks can simply disappear as unnecessary. We don't do those things any more. Some of them you will take up as your responsibility. Some can be left for hired help. But within the range of tasks that she can handle, let her and encourage her to do them. The kitchen tasks that she can still handle can become part of your new routine, or laundry, or cleaning, or fun stuff. She wants to contribute to the life of the family. Let her.

You both will know when fatigue sets in and it is just unwise to push any further. Help her out. That was true before the problem came into your lives. Identify those jobs that she can do and save them for her as is practical. She still wants to be useful, not just waited on.

7. ANTICIPATE THE CHANGES IN LIFESTYLE.

Again, every family has its own circumstances depending on the type of handicap or illness. There is quite a difference between an immobilized patient who is bedridden and one who can get around the house in a wheelchair or on foot with a walker or cane. The degree of mobility will govern a lot of the adaptations which are necessary to the house itself. There are experts at this who know the laws and the technical norms, so consult them or the documentation before proceeding with modifications to living quarters.

> ➤ The primary areas of concern relate to the patient's security, mobility, bathing, toilet access, sleeping, and meal preparation.

All over the house, try to look at the positions of furniture, the stairs, the equipment, the food, and all else in terms of her access to get to it and use it. What can be modified? What can no longer be accomplished? Talk these things over together without pressing for final decisions right away. Show a supportive and sympathetic attitude to help with acceptance of new limitations. Do this in stages as some tasks can be taken up after more healing and therapy. Others simply cannot be done any more. Be sensitive to the emotional dimensions of such decisions. Allow her to feel at home in her home.

8. GIVE YOURSELF SPACE TO GRIEVE.

While it is your spouse who suffered the major trauma, you have just been jerked around and turned inside out with no choice in the matter. You focus all your compassion on your fallen spouse, so your own pain as a person suffering major losses gets overlooked. Sure, your pain is small compared to your spouse, but it is real and it needs attention.

You can admit to yourself that you have been hurt too. Your roles have been redefined. Your plans have been upset. Your agenda has undergone a revolution. Your family life has been turned on its ear. Your future takes a new turn that you hardly understand and never asked for. You may need to balance home care with your normal employment. In some ways this is no different from missionaries going through culture shock as they adjust to a totally new environment which they barely understand and cannot control. Grow with it.

Because of the demands on caregivers it is not often practical to go off for a three-day retreat for prayer and analysis and planning. It's not going to happen. But just as the patient with the trauma has to go through a process of acceptance of the whole new way of life with unwanted limitations, the caregiver must also deal with his or her own new strictures. Life is just not the same any more. Some of that change is no fun at all.

You don't complain because your pain is just an inconvenience compared with what your spouse suffered. But you DO need to face up to your own need to adapt and adjust and accept some unwanted, unexpected, unwelcome roles in life. Our Father offers an inexhaustible supply of "grace to help in time of need," but it does not flow until caregivers admit that they have that need. Then the comfort comes. And you will need that many times.

For some people, grief is best expressed by talking it out with friends. For some, writing a journal is therapeutic. For others, a good workout in the gym or pool, or a long jog, helps clear the head and renew perspective. God is good. He is patient with our needs, and lets us find the various ways that we can deal with our new reality in his presence and be equipped to go on into a new life.

9. LEARN SOME LOGISTICS OF CAREGIVING.

Every kind of handicap or debilitating disease is different. There are no generic solutions. As your spouse works through the step-down treatments, you are in training. Much of the long-term care will take place at home after the formal treatment has been given in the hospital or therapy center. Watch closely and participate since you are the new therapist or nurses' aide once the patient is home.

Therapy. Be realistic about what you can expect to accomplish. You are not trained as a specialist in the many varieties of therapy, but will be instructed to follow up with your appropriate level of therapy. Part of therapy is to train family members to continue some of the healing routines which encourage restoration of mobility and control. Part of the new life is creating time to take the affected one to outpatient therapy at a nearby clinic. Be a part of that scene by enjoying the new circle of helpful friends and encouraging all who are involved in the rebuilding of life. Keep positive about it all.

Feeding. Learn about any special diet as to what must be included or avoided in the diet. Be sensitive to how much or little she can do for herself in preparing and serving food. Get beyond the humiliation of needing to be fed and just take it in stride as a part of your new life together. Let her do all that is possible, but don't hesitate to help as needed. Do not be embarrassed to cut her meat on her plate in a restaurant. Keep in mind that those who watch will admire the quality of your care for a loved one. Find and train others to help with feeding. There will be some accidents, so handle them with calm and good humor for the good of all. That handicap is not all there is to life, so talk about all the normal subjects at hand. Special matters come to be part of the "new normal."

Medications. Take charge of the scheduling of medications. Watch ahead as supplies on hand diminish and it is time to refill prescriptions without ever missing any days. Watch the prescriptions themselves as to when they run out, or call for another office visit or phone call for a new prescription. Keep the correct dosages on hand, whether in original containers or in the handy calendar boxes. Do it right. Some medications are dangerous and must be taken at the right time and frequency. This is your responsibility for a disabled patient. Keep abreast of anything that may affect the pacemaker by regular visits to the cardiologist or electrophysiologist. It ticks away faithfully.

Embarrassing Moments. People with disabilities have humiliating experiences of all sorts, and need calm rather than scorn or scolding. If there is partial paralysis it can affect the muscles that control elimination as well as those that control arm movements.

Caregivers learn to respond to occasional problems by creating an atmosphere of normalcy and acceptance as they get accustomed to dealing with problems and cleaning up afterward as needed. This is when love takes up the towel of service, and the caregiver senses the awkwardness of a situation which he would find humiliating. Seek to put the person at ease, to take it all in stride, and to stabilize the situation as readily as possible. Later on you can think and talk about how to communicate better to prevent some situations. Think ahead about travel situations to go at home first.

For a while we carried a small "emergency kit" in the van when we went out. It had some cleanup materials and a change of essential clothing. We rarely needed it, but it was a lifesaver when we did. It was a normal part of our routine.

When the patient gets upset it is time for the caregiver to take it with grace, knowing that all will calm down when the difficulty passes. Never let resentment build up after the emotion-laden crisis situations take place. The patient may express frustration with the caregiver when she is really angry at herself or her circumstances. Let it pass. You can take it. Be a man. Be her man, protective, honoring.

Travel. Handicaps complicate everything, especially travel. There may be extra luggage, a wheelchair, a walker, special equipment, exercise equipment, medications, hygiene supplies, spare clothing, and who knows what all. This is the new normal. Do not allow your spouse to just give up and stay home because "it is too much trouble to go out." She needs to know that you are quite willing to handle all of the extra stuff so she can enjoy getting out and around. Plan ahead for the extra time, extra stops, packing and repacking that come with the territory. Take it in stride. This is a dimension of your new existence as a caregiver and you will learn to welcome it.

Sleeping Arrangements. The special needs of the handicapped one now define where and how you both will sleep. You may well find yourselves in separate beds or even in separate rooms for your mutual good. That is fine. There is no law that a husband and wife must always occupy the same bed or room. Do what is right and best for your own circumstances, and don't worry about public opinion. The patient's sleeping setup will favor independence for getting to a bathroom with greatest ease, or to facilitate getting water or whatever else may be needed. It is common to have a monitor of the kind made for a baby nursery so the patient can call at any time. Get a one-way monitor so the casual noises from another room do not disturb her rest unnecessarily.

Emotional Sensitivity. Any kind of traumatic change in a person's life (serious car crash and injury, unsuccessful surgery, stroke, amputation, etc.) rubs nerves raw and causes emotional ups and downs. She is struggling to accept her new and unwelcome circumstances of dependency and weakness.

She has lost her freedom to move about, to choose her agenda, to be productive. The deep feelings attached to such changes do not pass in a few days or weeks. There is a long period of deep grieving which comes and goes from the level of awareness to underlying dread. Patients of such change often experience deep depression and despair, especially if there is no hope of supportiveness in the family. This is the time when a loving caregiver will allow his spouse to grieve freely, to express deep feelings, to find comfort in his acceptance and hugs and sympathy. Be clear that you are never embarrassed by her special needs. He will offer comfort from Scripture but not expect to use Bible verses as Band-Aids to fix everything in a few minutes. Patience is a valuable grace. Review the fruit of the Spirit (Galatians 5:22-23).

10. CARVE OUT YOUR OWN PERSONAL LIFE.

One of the biggest dangers for caregivers of spouses is becoming prisoners of their every whim. You must preserve your own balance and sanity and objectivity just so you can continue to care for her over the long haul. If you burn yourself out by being on duty 24/7 you will soon wallow in resentment and exhaustion and be of no use to anyone. You must decide whether to burn out in a few months, or learn to pace your involvement so you can keep at it for a lifetime. It is vitally important to maintain your own identity and have a life of your own outside the sickroom. You are still a whole person, not just an adjunct to the disabled one.

You need to get out with other people, with and without your spouse. You do need your own sense of freedom and initiative at times. The sickroom crowds in and clouds over, so you need the perspective of a clear sky and varieties of activities. You still need to stretch your mind and refresh your spirit. You have poured yourself out to meet those needs with your spouse, and do not dare run out of your own reserve.

If you spend all you have, you are then of no use to the very ones you seek to help. Build enough margin into your life to have a reserve of energy and creativity and emotional vitality that allows you to spring back when the times get really tough. You must preserve and renew yourself, even if only to continue to help your loved one. Don't get drained so dry that you become the next victim needing help. It's easy to do. When someone has fallen into a well, the rescuers do not jump into the well with him but stay near on firm ground where they can pull him out.

Keep up your own health. Someone else's illness or misfortune does not make your health problems go away. You won't get babied as much as before, but you need to keep healthy and fit, and keep any of your own illness away from your spouse at her most vulnerable times. Get help. Too many caregivers have neglected their own health because their spouses were so much worse off, and then had to face their own crises. Don't pretend you are well if you are not, both for your sake and the one you care for. Some treatments can wait a while, but some must be attended to right away. Take care of yourself or your loved one will not have a loving caregiver any more.

It is hard to take some time off and get away. It is hard to let others take your place for a while in the sickroom when you feel responsible to give the care that is needed. You cannot do it all, whether it is your spouse or yourself making such demands. Relax. A day or so away alone in a motel can be a lifesaver, or with a caring friend, or at a Bible conference. It is worth the cost. The fact that the patient cannot get away from the new condition does not mean that you cannot. You can, and must take time off.

In the midst of demanding ministry, Jesus commanded the disciples to "come apart for a while," probably before they came apart forever. Remember how Elijah overspent his spiritual and emotional budget to the point of suicidal depression? (Here we will read between the lines of 1Kings 19:1-8.) We would have expected God to call for long religious exercises of study and meditation and prayer. It would be time for introspection and repentance. No, God prescribed stranger things. He told Elijah to go off by himself, take a long nap, have a good meal, play a while, loaf some more, and just rest in God's fatherly embrace. Ahhhhhh!

Sometimes we caregivers need a bit of solitude like that.

Welcome to your new life as a caregiver. It is new, and it IS life, and it won't go away. You live out the loving life of Christ within you in new dimensions of service. Being a servant means allowing another's needs to set your agenda. Jesus did that. So can you. Sometimes it means letting Him do all of that caring through you. That takes the onus off you. Enjoy!

In my new role as a caregiver I have happily and proudly shared the stage with our daughter Margie. From the first day of discovery she has brought a level of maturity and insight into our process that has encouraged us all. This is not so much from having been a Psych major in college as being a sensitive and cheerful person who has faced her own challenges head-on. Now that she is a nurse her level of professionalism has risen to complement her caring spirit. Her other patients in the hospital get to enjoy that as well.

CHECK-UP: How are you measuring up? Most of us do not, at first, anyway. Think through your CHECKLIST FOR BETTER CAREGIVING. Or, write out your checklist if you have not done that already.

8.

THE LONG-TERM GAME

Stage 7: Lifelong Adaptation

The traumatic events of the stroke eventually enter the category of "history." The effects of the stroke are ever-present, but the stark emotional impact of the initial weeks has been tempered by experience. There is a new spice to life, salted with tears, peppered with problems, but going forward. Where do we go from here?

Let's look beyond the first year or two, bumpy with adjustments and learning curves. By that time many of the major decisions have been rendered, and the life of the family is settling into its new "normal."

As I write this, we have passed fifteen years since Doris' stroke. We are also into our middle 70s, so we remember that the simple effects of age complicate any analysis of stroke effects. I retired at the end of 2009 so it is a good time for me to be home full time now. Seven years of running two busy lives was plenty!

In our new "normal" I do most of the cooking, which I have long enjoyed, and the grocery shopping, which I have never enjoyed. Guys like machines, even when they are a washer and dryer, and Doris does most of the folding. We discovered that her folding goes well, until you add the extra dimension of sleeves on tee shirts. That kicks it up to a new level of topological complexity (my term, not hers) that makes tee shirts utterly incomprehensible. OK, I fold the shirts, no sweat. Doris has a friend with a home cleaning business clean our house the way she wants it cleaned (in contrast to how her hubby might muddle through it all). And that friend is also a pleasant companion so they minister to one another in their conversations. Doris generally manages the dishwasher which she can do from her wheelchair.

At one point Doris expressed her pleasant surprise at how readily I had risen to the occasion as a ready caregiver. I explained that I knew that if the tables were turned so that I was the patient, she would eagerly care for me. I just inwardly consulted with her and took my lessons from her on expressing love in serving.

Yes, there have been times when I have gotten quite tired of it all and just really told her off! My backlog of sour feelings can pour out in a rush. But I was always thankful afterward that I never did that when she was around. We have negotiated some elements of our new life, and learned a lot about mutual respect and clear communication. Some needs are immediate, and other matters can wait. We're both still learning, and always will be. There is no instruction manual except the one we write in our daily actions.

A leg brace makes it possible for Doris to walk. We've used this and that model, but it is still a leg brace, for her left leg (you knew that already). At first she hated the thing, but soon realized what a friend it was, enabling her to walk. She was struggling along with her walker in one rehab facility, and passed a lady in a wheelchair. She looked up at Doris and sighed, "It must be so nice to be able to walk!" Suddenly Doris felt privileged, young and spry. Perspective helps.

Her bed is still in the living room so she does not need to tackle the stairs in the morning and night when she is at her worst. It gives her easy access to the bathroom nearby. So at night there are occasional sounds of Velcro as that leg brace gets set aside for the remainder of the night. It is a happy reminder that she is independent in such personal care. She can pick out her own clothes and get dressed, except for her compression stockings which have become a normal part of our post-breakfast routine. She knows she can call for help at any time and I will come. The problem has been that I hear her call when she has not called. It may be my own tummy grumbling, or a bit of snoring (Moi?), or a Canada goose flying overhead. I go to her bedside and find her fast asleep. So we agree that if she is calling me she will call two times, once to waken me and once to call for my aid.

She began walking with a cane and occasionally used a walker, and now always uses a walker. In the house she is either in her recliner chair or whizzing around in her wheelchair, fussing when the carpet slows her down. That recliner chair is her command post with her iPad, her reading, her prayer lists, her TV remote, and her stack of catalogs from every mail order house in the country. The doctor insists that she walk instead of getting a power wheelchair, and Margie and I have held her to that. Years later when she faced minor surgery on her wrist we splurged and got her a lift chair to avoid putting pressure on the healing right wrist. It was time for that.

We did get a walk-in bathtub which has made it significantly easier for her to bathe independently, after a bit of setup on my part. With the railings on both sides of the stairs she grips confidently, climbs slowly, and only needs help negotiating the top step. Once there, she is pretty much on her own for the luxury of a nice warm bath. We have looked casually into a power chair for riding up and down stairs, probably our next project of that sort.

At one point the Benefits Manager at the mission came to my office with a card marked with a number well over $100,000. "Is this my new salary?" I asked amazed. "No, that is what the stroke has cost so far in what insurance has paid." We thanked the Lord for excellent insurance coverage so that our co-pay share was manageable. I suggested that some of the best medicine for Doris is an occasional steak dinner, and thought that therapeutic meals should be covered by the insurance. Well, he needed a good laugh that day.

One unexpected struggle of Doris' daily Bible reading was just lifting her large study Bible. Later she found the iPad program of Bible Gateway much easier to manage. We noticed how suffering can enhance spiritual sensitivity. She read in Isaiah 43:1-3, "But now, thus says the LORD, who created you,… 'Fear not, for I have redeemed you; I have called you by name; you are Mine. When you pass through the waters, I will be with you; and through the rivers, they shall not overflow you…For I am the LORD your God, the Holy One of Israel, your Savior.' " None of these trials are a surprise to Jesus, and He can sympathize having suffered Himself far worse than what we experience. So we hang on. He offers a sympathetic ear, as noted in Hebrews 4:15-16.

The one catastrophe all (of us) older folks dread is falling down. When bones get brittle, a fall can be a life-changer. Doris has had a few spills, both minor and major, but she has bounced back with remarkable endurance. A couple of times she looked like I had beaten her up since her anticoagulant encourages bruising.

One item of training at the therapy hospital was about how to get up after a fall, or even after exercising on the floor. We have practiced getting her up so we know what to expect. Hint: exercise on a bed rather than on the floor. So we have our slow getting-up routine once we check for pain and allow calm to return as needed. Doris can crawl, so we head for the couch and take off a cushion. She can kneel on the couch cushion to raise her up a bit, and then we get her good leg under her as we both lift and turn to sit on the couch. Pause for a breath, and go on with life. We have called friends to come help lift her up, and it is always possible to call an ambulance to get a pickup if she is just too tired out to make the effort. We resonated with a surgeon who was interviewed on TV about his early struggles, and he observed, "It doesn't get any easier, but you get used to how hard it is." Been there; done that.

Our calendar is remarkably full for a couple of old timers, but we plan ahead. With Doris' waning strength (well, ok, mine too) we plan half days of gentle activities for a day trip with a late start and early return. There are occasional concerts or movies or special church services or banquets that we enjoy at a pace she can handle. Will this be with wheelchair, or Rollator, or regular walker? On arrival anywhere I first spot the ladies' room and seek easy access to it.

The original vision loss left Doris without peripheral vision on the left side of both eyes. But with time and some therapeutic measures her vision returned to normal. She still consciously has to observe the left half of her universe, but that is becoming habitual. So the nagging question was whether she could drive again. Doris tooled around large stores in the power carts without incident, good sign. I took her out to an open parking lot and put her in the driver's seat to try a gentle run (since she did still have a valid driver's license). All went well in our trial run, and again.

So we inquired into the legal dimensions of driving and it was mostly a matter of clearance from her physician. Doris enrolled in special post-stroke driving lessons. But after only one lesson the teacher informed her that she did not need lessons, only a bit more practice for confidence and familiarity. But her driving skills were intact. The doctor favored her driving. When the time came for Doris to renew her license we would find out if the BMV was formally informed of the stroke to shut down driving privileges. We didn't ask but simply applied for a new license. No obstacle, new license in hand. She was free! Well, within sensible limits.

Since I was back on a regular work schedule, her being able to drive alone was a major release from being totally dependent on me or friends to get to a store. Now the major obstacles were her physical limitations of agility or stamina, but she had the option of getting out. I felt good that she exercised good sense about her limitations. A couple of times she backed out of the garage and just had to accept the fact that she was not really in good physical or emotional shape for driving that day, and pulled back inside. The town thanks you for wisdom. So with license in hand Doris returned to the roads, careful to check the left side, preferring quiet side streets, shunning the freeways. One more degree of freedom was a reality!

The time did come later, when the effects of age and the stroke were catching up with Doris, that Margie and I agreed that she should not renew her driver's license five years later. She agreed, but not without a further sense of loss and limitation. It was time.

When I was a young teenager I was the baker in our family. So when it came time for me to just take charge of the kitchen, the shopping, and most meal preparation I was favorably inclined. The need to be the main cook did not make a haute cuisine chef of me, but I did need to provide good and interesting meals for our little family. At times Margie said, "I'll fix dinner tomorrow." I was always glad since she is a far better and more imaginative cook than I will ever be. My goal was to have about thirty essential dinners that I could confidently prepare in rotation. It is all easier during grilling season. It was a helpfully realistic limitation on a new responsibility.

We travel less now, but even when we visit family we find it best to get a motel room. That gives us our own retreat whenever we need to just disappear for a while without inconveniencing anyone else. Doris needs more sleep than I do, so in the morning I go eat breakfast and read a while, and then bring breakfast for her to munch at her own convenience. Every family has its own routines. About the only early activity is Sunday morning when we should be out the door by 8:45. For most families that is late, but we avoid scheduling early events.

In the aftermath of the stroke, Doris and I have flown to south Brazil to be with family two times. The trip in 2003 was tougher than our return in 2007, but proved that she is not a prisoner at home. Our new handicaps are not the end of sensible adventures. Were there many difficulties? Of course, but none that prevented the trips to see our grandchildren in their life setting, and the dear folks at their church who had prayed so much for us. Doris was among them as a real answer to their prayers. Dave managed to rent an antique wheelchair for our use from the veterans' home. What a contraption! But it got us around where we needed to go. We came to deeply appreciate the laws in our own land that call for wheelchair accessibility more deeply implemented here, while just getting well underway in Brazil.

Our real adventure was a long-time dream. We went out to the West Coast by train! For real?? Leg 1: Cleveland to Chicago. Leg 2: Chicago via St. Louis and Albuquerque to Los Angeles. Leg 3: Los Angeles to Portland where we spent a delightful week with Doris' western family. Leg 4: the northern route from Portland to Chicago. Note to self: you do NOT see the glory of the Rocky Mountains when you pass through at 4am! Leg 5: Chicago to Cleveland. What made it work so well was that Amtrak's passenger cars each have a handicap suite that spans the width of the car, and has a private bathroom. What made it difficult was the swaying that made walking the halls virtually impossible for Doris. So we had the fine meals brought to our suite and we just enjoyed having the countryside come to us through the large windows on both sides of the train. There are some things we just can't do, but plenty that we can do. The handicap suite cost less than coach fare. And my ticket was just half of Doris' since I went as the caregiver. Nice! The whole circuit was two enjoyable, tiring weeks, worth the effort even while we were glad to get home. It was a wonderful trip, and we are glad we tackled it – once.

All this is just to say we have come to make some simple allowances for our needs and we continue to LIVE. There are many days when Doris is content just to be home for the day. We can sense when she is tired out and just needs more help with routine matters like changing clothes. She can sense when I have gotten to the end of my tether and it is better for her to do more things for herself.

We have learned to keep Doris' blood sugar on an even keel since it seems to directly affect her emotional agility. A sweet tweedly song on her smartphone alarm reminds us not to delay lunch too long, so Alice in Wonderland does not morph into the Queen of Hearts. Every family learns its own little ways of creating a coping culture for joy. But our life is not disability, but abilities. It is our life, together, and both of us give a little here and there to help it go smoothly.

We have learned that grieving the loss of one's freedom just does not evaporate. Talking about it is far more healing than stuffing it inside somewhere to fester. Just confining frustration into words helps to keep it in perspective as a shrinking part of our larger life. But talking presumes that someone cares to listen. One way that a spouse can express love is to listen and warmly welcome the release, without letting the venting escalate into an eruption. Small tremors prevent major earthquakes by accommodating inner tension and relieving it before it can accumulate to a serious bursting point. Anger is not sin, though we can manage it in unrighteous ways. Allow the expression of honest feelings with realism. That fosters objectivity and calm.

We are both cancer survivors, and have enjoyed a full life of service to God and people, so we fold the stroke into our packet of life circumstances and continue to roll, at our own pace. I have learned that a woman's work is never done, especially when entrusted to a mere man!

It is hard to be angry at God for allowing such tragedy to crash into our lives when we are regularly reading His Word. The Bible stories and the Psalms and Epistles are not merely a distraction from the hard present reality. The reading is a conversation with a loving Father who has made promises and has a great track record for keeping them, whether to His nation, His church, or His people. There are songs that express that Word in terms that resonate with our hurts and questions. When Doris was down she loved to listen to *You Are Still Holy* as sung by Kim Hill.

Holy, You are still holy
Even when the darkness surrounds my life.
Sovereign, You are still sovereign
Even when confusion has blinded my eyes.

Lord, I don't deserve Your kind affection
When my unbelief has kept me from Your touch.
I want my life to be a pure reflection
Of Your love.
    And so I come into Your chamber,
    And I dance at Your feet, Lord.
    You are my Savior
    And I'm at Your mercy.
    All that has been in my life
    Up 'til now,
    It belongs to You.
    You are still Holy.

Holy, you are still holy,
Even though I don't understand your ways.
Sovereign, You will be sovereign,
Even when my circumstances don't change

Lord, I don't deserve Your tender patience
When my unbelief has kept me from Your truth.
I want my life to be a sweet devotion...To You

And so I come into Your chamber,
And I dance at Your feet, Lord.
You are my Savior
And I'm at your mercy.
All that has been my life
Up 'til now
It belongs to You.
I belong to You.

You are still holy.
You are still sovereign.
You are still holy, Lord.
You are still righteous.
You are all-knowing
You are still holy.

By Rita Springer,   Sung by Kim Hill in the CD *Arms of Mercy*,
StarSong Records (Sparrow Group) 1998 © 1998 Mercy Publishing.

The stroke brought other decisions to the fore. What activities will she NOT be able to continue? This question accompanied any retirees' normal need to cut back, trim down, give away, and toss out the accumulated detritus of decades of typical life. We had been sorting our stuff rather than leave it for the kids to do for us. Quilting? Nope. Sewing? Not really. Cooking? Less and less (but the new chef still needs the old pots and pans since we have hardly given up eating). Reading? More than ever, particularly when prime-time TV offers so much drivel.

I conclude with a few general observations about life after a stroke.

Grief lasts. A stroke is akin to death. It doesn't end the life of one in its grasp, but can so limit his or her life that there is a partial death. The post-stroke life has losses of freedoms and options and skills that may provoke occasional grieving for many years. Some people can shrug things off readily. Good for them. But many people remember how it was, and pine for the past, even in healthy remembrance. After a major stroke, or other life-altering event, you do not just feel bad for a year and then live happily ever after. The grieving goes on, and on, and on. Grief ebbs and returns, but is never gone. Real living calls for focus outside the sickroom.

Caregivers and other friends need to allow such grief, but not allow it to overwhelm the patient. It is not wrong to be sad about lost abilities, any more than to grieve the loss of deceased loved ones. But it is unhealthy to sink into depression and despair when one's focus is on the past rather than on the future. Wellness is in the mind as much as in the body.

Emotional needs are real. We wonder if the compression of one's physical life is compensated for in the expansion of the emotional life. If we can't run and jump physically we may respond to our world with more profound emotions about our smaller universe, our more limited control, our curtailed participation. Feelings need to be expressed, and heard, with respect.

After years, the patient's emotional palette may become more limited, so that anger plays a larger role in his or her expression. There is less emotional agility, and less restraint on just speaking one's mind whether or not it is considerate. It is said that one function of the frontal lobe is inhibition, the ability to weigh the propriety of one's thoughts before lobbing them into the public or family arena. If so, that function may be reduced, calling for understanding.

One way or another, the person suffering the stroke needs a measure of patience as to any tweaking of the personality or emotional expressiveness. The family wants to provide an environment of security and welcome, but not indulging every whim that may poison life for others.

Caregiving is an expression of love. A traumatic event like a stroke can divide a couple if each is focused on his or her own needs. A loving bond in marriage absorbs the strains of adversity so the couple can share the pain and effort to survive and even prosper. YES, there IS life after a stroke! Yes, there IS love after a stroke even as it takes on new forms and activities. Spending more time together becomes a benefit rather than a trial, even granting normal times of privacy for each one. Both husband and wife need to maintain loving attitudes, civility in the asking and giving of help, and mutual respect.

Depression can be dangerous. A common long-term response to a stroke is depression, hopelessness, and awareness that there will be no going back to the familiar "normal." Some may have been prone to depression before the stroke, only to have it made worse. For some, the stroke may mess with the output of their body's natural pharmacy, the God-given production of hormones and other chemical messengers that affect one's emotional well-being. It is good to include consultation with mental health professionals when there are signs of depression beyond some normal discouragement. Sometimes we need to supplement our internal natural pharmacy with pills that keep the emotional balance that feeds good health.

A deeper sense of loss and hopelessness can lead to the desire to just end the agony and take one's own life to stop being a bother to so many people. Any such expressions of suicidal thoughts must be taken seriously. Family members can sense a shift from a healthy longing for Heaven into a darker sense of despair that might impel one to take steps to speed that transition along. Talk, and listen. Allow the patient to express herself without imposing judgments beyond helpful comfort. If there is reason for serious concern, call for help from your pastor, physician, or counselor.

Spiritual health is vital. While Doris' circle of physical activity has been drastically reduced, her engagement in spiritual growth has been vigorous. Her iPad allows interaction with missionary friends around the world, and brings a daily Bible reading plan to read through the Bible in a year. My retirement has allowed us to enjoy more leisurely time every morning for Bible reading and prayer together, reflecting on what is going on around the world and in our areas of personal interest. We have enjoyed simply being together for much of the day as a normal lovey-dovey couple. And we both have our solo activities that occupy us separately.

A robust relationship with Jesus Christ turns our focus away from our own problems to see a needy world from God's perspective and be involved in prayer and giving and encouragement. That is not so much an antidote for depression as a preventative measure, and a way of life. Part of that health is access to friends and to live church services with the smiles and hugs and interaction that TV church cannot provide.

THANK YOU for letting us share our story. It is not over yet. Whatever is good about it began long before the stroke struck. New tragic circumstances do not turn a dysfunctional family into a smooth and peacefully operating one. New tragic circumstances need not turn a functional family into one that has become dysfunctional. Start early working on that one. Look for the positive elements of your own circumstances so you are not defined by new limitations.

CHECK-UP: What adjustments and improvements do you foresee in YOUR case? What advice will you give to others who experience a stroke or similar disabling condition?

9.

READ FOR GROWTH

This is not the bibliography for our little book. It is a review of some of the many books on today's market that encourage both patients and caregivers. The entire family suffers when one member suffers a stroke or any other major debilitating illness or injury with long-term aftereffects. Read others' stories; you are NOT alone. Share this story with others.

The purpose of this simple work has been to invite you to a conversation about our experience as a family in the aftermath of Doris' stroke. When we are devastated by a major tragedy of any sort we hardly know where to turn or what to ask. Some can offer medical explanations, while others major on spiritual comfort. We have sought to integrate these fields with an emphasis on the spiritual dimensions of struggles to recover what was lost. Our focus has not been religion in a generic sense, but our personal reliance on Jesus Christ as our Savior and Friend. The reality of our faith in Christ was tested and found to be a resource of inestimable value. The value is not in our faith, but in the object of our faith, Christ Himself. Having that bedrock of spiritual reality already in place as the core of our lives and our home kept our rocking ship from sinking.

The books listed here give a similar Evangelical perspective. There are plenty of other good works that focus on the medical layer, or the social layer, or the family layer, or the emotional recovery layer of surviving a major health event. Our list complements that with books that address the specifically spiritual layer of our experiences in the context of all the other layers. They ALL need to be addressed in the aftermath of tragedy. Few of these works deal with strokes, but offer valuable models for coping with various sorts of maladies that attack us, whether or not we are Bible-believing Christians.

Arthur, Kay
> 1997 *As Silver Refined: Learning to Embrace Life's Disappointments.* Colorado Springs: Waterbrook Press / Random House. This well-regarded Bible teacher deals with stress, pain, discouragement, and despair for restoration of spirit by the Spirit.

Chapman, Mary Beth with Ellen Vaughn
> 2010 *Choosing to SEE.* Grand Rapids MI: Revell division of Baker Publishing. A mom full of the pain of loss opens her heart to share how Jesus works in us in those awful times of disappointment, depression, and questioning. This is an adventure of tears for any family that suffers a devastating event, to survive intact.

McQuilkin, J. Robertson.
> 1998 *A Promise Kept.* Wheaton IL: Tyndale House. The former president of a Christian college explores the changes brought by his beloved wife's descent into Alzheimer's disease, and accepts caring for her as a ministry for the Lord they loved together. This is a beautiful love story and a model for the caregiver's spiritual attitude.

Tada, Joni Eareckson
> 1997 *When God Weeps.* Grand Rapids: Zondervan. Subtitled "Why our sufferings matter to the Almighty," Joni's sensitive work encourages those trapped in handicaps of all sorts.
> 2003 *The God I Love: A Memoir.* Grand Rapids: Zondervan. Joni relates her personal pilgrimage with Christ as a quadriplegic for several decades, finding comfort and purpose in God's redesign for her life and ministry.

Talley-Cunningham, Marian
> 2004 *The Faces of Grief:* A Women's Bible Study. Greenville SC. BJU Press/JourneyForth. This pastor's wife, and grief counselor at a local funeral home, writes of God's comfort in the Scriptures both before and after the passing of her two beloved husbands. She learned by experience how Christ turns crippling sorrow into profound hope.

Thompson, Douglas K.
> 2003 *Refuge from the Storm.* Caring for a loved one with a terminal illness. Fairfax VA: Xulon Press. ISBN 1-591603-97-8. Doug recorded his deep feelings in prose and poetry as his beloved wife was failing with Alzheimer's disease for a decade.

Yancey, Phillip
  1977   *Where is God when it Hurts?* Grand Rapids: Zondervan. A
         pastor explores pain and its messages to us from God, not just for
         coping but for reconstructing joyful life.
  1991   *Disappointment with God.* New York: Harper Paperbacks (or
         Zondervan 1988). At times God seems silent. How do we make
         contact, draw closer, get through obstacles of doubt to enjoy Him
         again?

MEET THE AUTHOR

Bill Smallman was a mechanical engineer, pastor, missionary in Brazil, mission administrator, professor, editor and writer. He has taught in 27 nations. But for this book he is a happy husband, father, and caregiver, a career for which his titles like Rev., or Dr., have no relevance now in retirement. Bill and Doris married in 1962, and enjoy their son and daughter, and their three grandchildren. The suburbs of Cleveland, Ohio, have been home to them since 1980. Bill has degrees in Mechanical engineering, Theology, Communications, and a doctorate in Cross-Cultural Ministry. He has authored or edited a number of books that are readily located on Amazon.Com by entering the author name as either Bill Smallman or William Smallman to find different books.

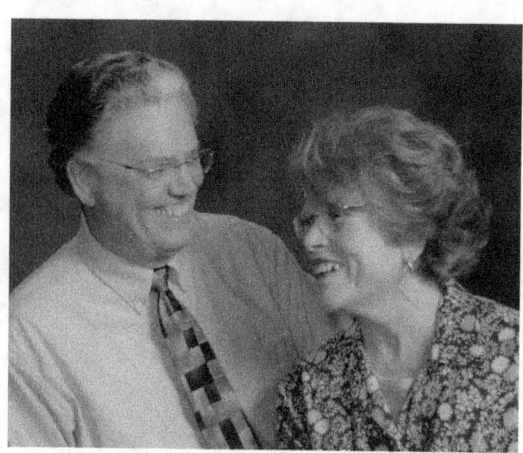

www.ingramcontent.com/pod-product-compliance
Lightning Source LLC
Chambersburg PA
CBHW062049280526
45788CB00003B/1167